STEPHEN HOLT M.D.
PROVIDES NATURAL PATHWAYS
TO HEALTHY SLEEP

WITH

THE SLEEP NATURALLY PLAN™

COMBAT INSOMNIA WITHOUT DRUGS, USING LIFESTYLE CHANGES AND NUTRITIONAL SUPPORT FOR SLEEP

Foreword by Eric R. Braverman M.D.

www.sleepnaturally.com
www.wellnesspublishing.com
www.naturesbenefit.com

For Information Only: Call 1-973-824-8800

www.wellnesspublishing.com

 Editorial, sales and distribution rights and permissions inquiries should be addressed to : Wellness Publishing, 105 Lock Street, Suite 405, Enterprise Development Center, NJIT, Newark, NJ 07103.

Book cover design: Asha Azhar
Book layout: Jonathan Gullery.

Manufactured in United States.
Library of Congress Cataloging-in-Publication Data.
Holt, Stephen 1950 –

Title: "Sleep Naturally"

ISBN – 0-9714224-7-8

1. Sleep 2. Hypnotic Drugs 3. Alternative Medicine 4. Healthy Sleep 5. Dietary Supplements 6. Lifestyle 7. Sleeping pills 8. Side effects of sleep drugs 9. Nutritional Support for Sleep

CONTENTS

FOREWORD 7
ERIC R. BRAVERMAN, M.D.

PREFACE 9
STEPHEN HOLT, M.D.

CHAPTER 1
UNDERSTANDING SLEEPLESSNESS 13

CHAPTER 2
SLEEPING, DREAMING AND BIOLOGICAL CLOCKS 32

CHAPTER 3
THE SCIENCE OF SLEEP 47

CHAPTER 4
HEALTH CONSEQUENCES OF LACK OF SLEEP 61

CHAPTER 5
A LITANY OF SLEEP AIDS 77

CHAPTER 6
SLEEP NATURALLY: NUTRITIONAL SUPPORT FOR NATURAL SLEEP 91

CHAPTER 7
THE SLEEP NATURALLY PLAN 112

REFERENCES 119

ABOUT THE AUTHOR 123

A Note to the Reader

The author of this book is not attempting to provide advice on the treatment or prevention of disease. While the health benefits of dietary supplements are reviewed, it is not the intention of the author to provide an alternative to orthodox physician/patient relationship. Rather, it is the objective of the author to expand the dimensions of orthodox medicine by providing more interest in remedies of natural origin. Food is being incorporated more into medical practices in the 21st century, where diet and lifestyle will play a dominant role in preventive medicine. This book was not written to endorse the use of specific products for any treatment purpose. The conclusions in this book represent the author's opinions of medical, scientific, folkloric and lay writings on the various topics discussed.

The publisher and author accept no responsibility for the use of any agents mentioned in this book. Before any individual self-medicates, he or she is advised to seek the advice of a qualified healthcare professional. The author does not support unsubstantiated claims of health benefits of foods or dietary supplements. This book must not be interpreted as product labeling.

www.wellnesspublishing.com

FOREWORD

Dr. Stephen Holt, M.D. FACP, FRCP (C), MRCP (UK), FACG, FACN, FACAM requires no introduction to the dietary supplement industry or the modern movement of Alternative and Complementary Medicine. His name reverberates with respect for his work in natural medicine on an international basis. This book is an example of Dr. Holt's many contributions to natural pathways to health, where he tackles the natural therapeutics of sleep with "SLEEP NATURALLY".

Tens of millions of Americans cannot get a "good night's sleep." These sleep-deprived individuals may reach for a variety of drugs that have short-term benefits, with long-term disadvantages. The brain is not easily fooled by a simple chemical that may focus on a relatively distinct and small number of tissue receptors. The health costs of side effects from drugs used for sleep are a major problem. This problem is underexplored in medicine and the use of over-the-counter sleeping drugs is a particular concern. To seek alternative approaches with safe and effective approaches to gain restful sleep has become a major health initiative for the nation. This approach is well described in this book.

Poor sleep means poor health. Dr. Holt's account of the physical and mental consequences of sleep deprivation is presented in a manner for everyone to understand. This book is loaded with good advice on changes in lifestyle and behavior that can restore sleep rhythms for the insomniac. Dr. Holt discusses new findings in sleep science, but he probes early research on sleep to rediscover natural, effective approaches to good sleep.

Dr. Holt is best known for his talent in using remedies of natural origins for disease or disorder management. In this book, he addresses the logic of leading-edge dietary supplement technology in the development of natural formulas for sleep. Using the precedent of the safety and efficacy of several herbs and nutrients, Dr. Holt describes the concepts of synergy. The use of synergy in formulations takes balanced doses of natural substances to achieve a desired effect in sleep promotion. Each component of a synergistic formula adds to the overall desired effect. Dr. Holt provides new creative ideas of adding to our natural sleep armamentarium, which includes 5 Hydroxytryptophan, Melatonin, B Vitamins and other alternatives, such as the Cranial Electrical Stimulation (CES) device. I enjoy working with Dr. Holt in his continuing attempt to contribute to the "sleep natural feel" with sleep formulas that are natural and do not produce hangovers. Dr. Holt has sought to use "adaptogenic", natural substances, which not only induce hypnosis, but they also help balance body functions for health.

This book is well written in Dr. Holt's classic teaching style. The writings are excellent reading for the restless and anxious Americans who fight their relationships with the obligatory body function of sleep. Americans must thank Dr. Holt for his advice which may enrich people's waking and sleeping experiences. This book is a "must-read" for those people who are encumbered by lack of sleep, poor sleep or other sleep disorders.

Eric R. Braverman
Physician, New York
Best-selling Author
August 2003

PREFACE

One cannot take sleep for granted. Modern research has uncovered the importance of restful sleep in the prevention and management of many diseases. On an annual basis, as many as 100 million Americans may be troubled with difficulty in falling asleep, staying asleep or early morning awakening. This sleeplessness has precipitated an unfortunate and unhealthy reflex response from more than 30 million Americans that involves the taking of drugs to help sleep – a "quick fix" approach. This book describes the disadvantages and limitations of "the drug approach" and highlights the dangerous use or misuse of over-the-counter pharmaceuticals for sleep. There are many natural pathways to healthy sleep and these represent "first-line options" for the vast majority of people (about 65 million Americans) who suffer from insomnia.

Sleep science has emerged with newfound importance in modern medicine, such that there are thousands of physicians who specialize in sleep disorders. These experts in sleep direct a large number of newly developed "sleep centers" that are part of almost every community hospital; and these assessment and treatment facilities have emerged as "free-standing" outpatient sleep centers. These centers of medical excellence are accredited by government agencies that set standards for the diagnostic evaluation of sleep problems. While such medical facilities are relevant to people with more severe types of sleep disturbances or specific sleep conditions (e.g. narcolepsy or sleep apnea), they are outside the reach of the "average insomniac." Self-education and self-management of sleep disorders are emerging as an important public health initiative. Evidence exists that modern medicine is only accessing the tip of the iceberg when it comes to the management of sleep disorders and their social, medical and mental consequences.

Change in lifestyle, from adverse to positive habits, is the cornerstone of modern sleep management and this is a key focus of my recommendations. The premature use of prescription drugs, or OTC drugs, for sleeping must be considered unwise and even potentially dangerous. There are many nutritional agents that have a long history of use to allay anxiety and support sleep. The pharmaceutical revolution of the 20th century has tended to overshadow the real value of natural nutritional support for healthy sleep. This book describes the rational use of herbs, botanicals and nutrients for the promotion of sleep. Behavioral and lifestyle changes with the use of natural substances to promote healthy sleep may do more to solve the common sleep problems of the nation than the development of another "me-too" hypnotic (sleeping) drug.

Stephen Holt, M.D. August 2003

THE SLEEP NATURALLY PLAN™

Chapter 1:

UNDERSTANDING SLEEPLESSNESS

The Notion of Sleep Naturally

Many Americans crave a good night's sleep. Why some people sleep like a baby and others may wrestle in their beds depends upon a whole host of different factors. Environmental, social and medical issues can interrupt or promote sleep. Sleep is responsible for recuperation. Specific physical and mental regenerations occur during slumber; and without a "good night's sleep," well-being and health cannot prevail. Modern scientists continue to argue about the definition of good sleep, but sleep patterns and duration change dramatically with age, selected lifestyles and environmental factors.

So common is the inability to fall asleep or achieve sustained sleep, that there are thousands of different sleeping aids on the market. Anything ranging from comfortable clothing through to dangerous and addictive drugs are variably adopted by the American public to combat insomnia. The importance of sleep for health has become a major public health initiative in recent times. Practical applications of the science of sleep are now practiced in specialized "Sleep Centers" that have sprung up in every community hospital in the nation.

Previously somewhat ignored in medical practice, the body function of sleep is now foremost in the minds of many medical practitioners. For hospitals, pharmaceutical companies and manufacturers of bedroom contents, sleep is big business. Population studies have shown the magnitude of the negative impacts of poor sleep on the nation. In fact, insomnia causes great economic, social, physical and psychological problems. It causes the nation billions of dollars in poor job performance, traffic accidents and ill health.

This book examines first-line, safe and gentle options to promote healthy sleep. The notion that one can "**Sleep Naturally**" is of major appeal to about 100 million Americans who have developed a poor relationship with the cherished gift of sleep. While drugs and surgery may play a role in a small number of people with chronic sleep problems, natural approaches to healthy sleep must be preferred. In order to combat insomnia, this book reviews much information about natural methods that can be effective in the induction of safe and appropriate somnolence.

How to Evaluate Sleep?

There are many ways to evaluate the quality and duration of sleep. Insomnia can present itself with difficulty in falling asleep, disrupted sleep or early morning wakening. Many people with insomnia complain that they are not refreshed by sleep. It is quite important to define how long sleep problems may have been present. Chronic insomnia is defined as a condition that lasts longer than a month or so. There are many people who have experienced variable difficulty in sleeping for many years. In contrast, short-lived or transient insomnia usually lasts a few days and it is commonly precipitated by periodic stressful life events, such as travel or emotional upheavals. The "sleep history" is the most important way of assessing the characteristics of sleep disturbances. Table 1 is a helpful guide to questions that can be self-administered by questionnaire or by interview.

Questions for a Sleeping Partner

Do you wake up to your bed partner's snoring? (a clue to sleep apnea)
Does your bed partner seem to have trouble breathing at times? (a sign of sleep apnea)
Does your bed partner kick or jerk during sleep?

Questions on Daytime Sleep Patterns

What time do you wake up on work days, weekends and vacations?
Do you use an alarm clock to help you wake up in the morning?
Do you feel rested upon waking up?
Do you wake up with a headache or feeling like you have a hangover?
Do you feel tired during the daytime?
Do you take a nap? How long is your nap and what time?
Do you fall asleep during daytime?

Questions on Nighttime Sleep Patterns

What time do you retire at night?
Do you go to bed sleepy?
How long does it take you to fall asleep?
Do you sleep soundly through the night?
Have you been told that you snore?
Have you been told that you move in your sleep?

Table 1: Questions that can be asked of an individual who experiences sleep disturbance, together with questions that provide collateral information from others. This table is modified from Neubauer DN et al "Sleep Disorders", Chapter 85 in Principles of Ambulatory Medicine, Fourth Edition, Editors, Randol Barker et al, Williams and Wilkins, Baltimore, MD, 1994. The significance of these questions is covered by information in several sections of this book.

Sleep Impacts Health

Without sleep, health is lost. In contrast, poor health may cause insomnia. Several proverbs link health with good sleeping habits, supporting the adage: "The beginning of health is sleep." Gender differences exist in sleep habits. While women may complain more about sleep problems, several scientific studies imply that sleep in men is often of lower quality than it is in women. Furthermore, snoring is more common in men, but many women snore especially as they age. There may be some simple explanations for the reported discrepancy in snoring occurrence between men and women. Women tend to live longer than men and elderly women may not have a partner with whom to share or report their snoring. There is little doubt that men snore louder than women and their snoring symphonics may drown the noise of the snoring female.

Insomnia or snoring must be taken seriously if it is associated with breathing difficulties, excessive daytime sleepiness, morning headaches, interference with mental functioning or waking up with a lack of a refreshed feeling. Snoring may be a sign of sleep-related breathing disorders, such as sleep apnea. Sleep apnea is a significant disorder where an individual may periodically stop breathing at certain times of the night. People who snore and have symptoms of sleep deprivation should consider an evaluation by an expert in a sleep center. There are several common causes of persistent insomnia (Table 2)

Psychiatric illness	Chronic medical illness
Brain disease	Disturbances of Circadian Rhythm
Medications	Environmental and behavioral factors
Substance and drug abuse	Specific sleep disorders

Table 2: Some causes of long-standing insomnia.

The Elusive Sleep

About 100 million Americans can't sleep well. Many do not get the right amount of sleep, and some get their shuteye under the most unlikely conditions. Embarrassment occurs when sleep is unheralded or not welcome. We are all aware of people nodding off during a church service or while engaged in monotonous tasks. However, there are circumstances where unwanted sleep or drowsiness can be extremely dangerous. These circumstances include driving a vehicle, operating machinery, looking after kids or supervising important daily missions.

Formerly, society tended to ignore sleeplessness and so did many health care givers. To dismiss unwanted somnolence as behavior that is an inevitable part of a busy person's lifestyle is often a mistake. Lack of sleep is a major public health issue that is often unreported to health care professionals and it often goes undiagnosed or misdiagnosed. One can witness the symptoms and signs of sleep disturbances everyday. When unwanted sleep interferes with physical and social functions, an alarm bell should ring. Modern research is drawing our attention increasingly to the underestimated dangers of poor sleep patterns.

About 65 million Americans are believed to be insomniacs. Insomnia may be accepted by many people who lead a stressful lifestyle, but poor sleep is a serious public health problem. In fact, recent research indicates that poor sleep patterns may be associated with premature disability and death. In contrast, individuals who have adequate amounts of restful sleep are known to be healthier and they may live longer.

There are alarming trends reported in National Health Statistics. The casualties caused by driving while impaired with drowsiness from poor sleep or substance abuse, or both, are increasing in number. Poor sleep contributes to accidents in the workplace and many people are being labeled inappropriately with a diagnosis of chronic fatigue syndrome, when the real problem rests in sleep disorder. Individuals who complain of sleepiness during the day often present themselves with a variety of complaints. (Table 3)

Drowsiness	Inability to concentrate
Poor memory function	Passive or aggressive behavior
Lack of motivation	"Blues" or frank depression
General fatigue	Accidents in all locations

Table 3: Symptoms expressed commonly by people who are sleep deprived.

Sleep Deprivation is Linked to Common Disease

Elegant research shows that sleep disorders contribute to several chronic diseases, including the modern epidemics of heart disease, Syndrome X and maturity onset diabetes mellitus. Syndrome X is the combination of obesity, high blood pressure and high blood cholesterol, all linked by insulin resistance, with compensatory increases in blood insulin levels (Holt S, "Combat Syndrome X, Y and Z...", Wellness Publishing, Newark, NJ, 2002)

The importance of good sleep crosses all social, political, medical, legal and economic boundaries. Insomnia has bred new professions, including an increasing number of physicians who specialize in the management of sleep disorders and even an increasing number of lawyers who litigate sleep-related accidents and the adverse consequences of the side effects of sleep-inducing drugs.

Public Perceptions of Insomnia

Why some people are able to sleep with ease, whereas others despair from lack of sleep has puzzled humanity for ages. How much sleep one needs varies from one person to another. There are some who believe they have little need for it and get by on 4 to 5 hours, and those who feel they need 8 or more hours of sleep to fully recharge their body and mind. The duration and quality of a healthy person's sleep tends to diminish with age. A newborn baby can sleep for up to 17 hours per day, whereas the elderly are often restricted to 6 hours of sleep. Just what constitutes the normal duration of sleep is open to interpretation and definitions of normal sleep must occur in ranges, rather than absolute terms; and they must take into account the quality of sleep.

Sleep is Actually a State of Wakefulness for the Brain

Scientific studies in the 1950s revolutionized the way scientists view sleep. Fifty years ago, Dr. H. W. Magoun, M.D. and his colleagues described the presence of arousal mechanisms in the brain. It is the activation of these arousal mechanisms that causes wakefulness, rather than the inhibition of brain functions that is involved in sleep. These days, the sleeping and waking mechanisms of the human brain are subject to evolving stresses, the consequences of poor nutrition, excessive fatigue and even environmental pollutants. In addition, brain mechanisms that control sleep are often "drugged" with pharmaceuticals and under these circumstances they may not function to provide restful sleep.

The discovery of rapid eye movements (REM) during sleep and the clear definition of sleep cycles, related to biorhythms, have resulted in major expansions in knowledge about fitful sleep. This knowledge has led scientists to understand several effective ways to get necessary "shut-eye". The general public still seems to regard sleep as a state of stupor or quiescence where inactivity prevails. However, sleep is a process of major activity within the body, where the brain is involved in much turbulent activity. Sleep has become a great medical frontier to investigate. Understanding healthy sleep provides a source of key information about body structures and functions that are responsible for general well-being.

Monitoring the Body During Sleep

The study of symptoms and signs of people with abnormal sleep can be linked to elegant recordings of brain electrical activity (electroencephalographic, EEG recordings). In addition, changes in body functions, such as breathing, heart function and muscle function, can be monitored during sleep. Such sleep studies have illuminated changes in body functions that can occur during mental illness, heart disease, asthma and even odd events, such as sleepwalking.

The EEG and the study of eye movements using an apparatus called "oculogram" provide measurements that characterize the celebrated five stages of sleep. The five stages of sleep begin with stages 1 and 2 of light slow-wave sleep, followed by stages 3 and 4 of delta sleep characterized by electrical activity in the brain. The final phase, or stage 5, is a deep form of sleep, characterized by rapid eye movements (REM). Figure 1 is modified from an article published more than thirty years ago by Kales A. et al. (Ann Intern Med 68:1078, 1968). This figure is reproduced to illustrate how active and changing brain and selected muscle functions are during different stages of sleep (Figure 1). Clearly, few would disagree with the notion that sleep consists of multiple periods of considerable activity for the brain and body. The recordings of the brain and body during sleep have become very sophisticated in recent times.

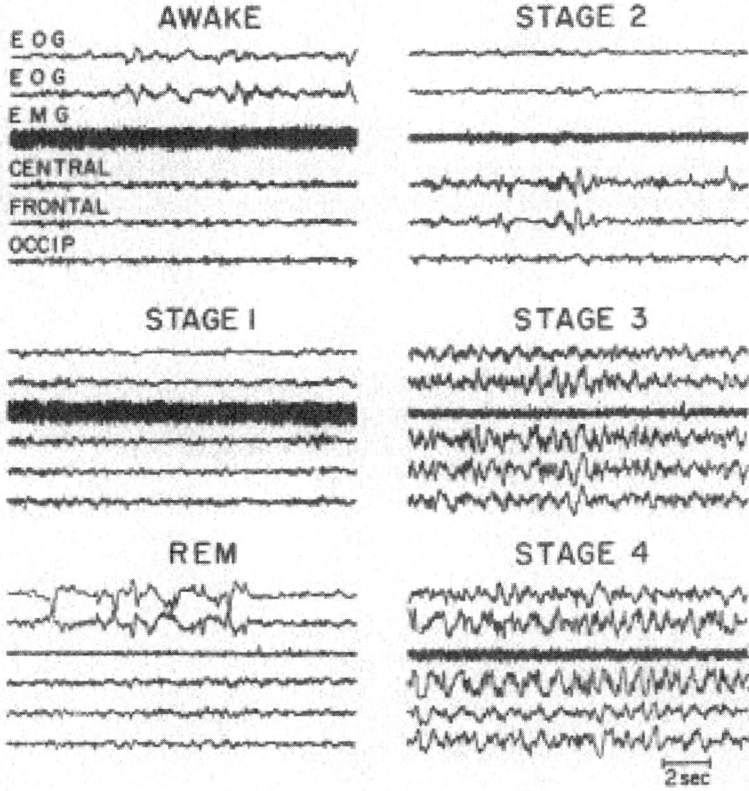

Figure 1: The 6 groups of recordings show changes in eye movements with an electrooculogram (EOG), muscle movements with an electromyogram (EMG) and electroencephalographic recordings from different areas of the head, front, center and rear, i.e., frontal, central and occipital (OCCIP) regions, respectively. Recordings are very active from the EMG and EOG during wakefulness, but examination of stage 3 and 4 sleep shows rapid eye movements (REM). These patterns of eye movement, muscle function and brain electrical activity are quite fascinating, even to the lay person. (Modified from Kales et al, Ann Intern Med 68:1078, 1968)

Cycles of Sleep

Over a period of 24 hours, patterns of sleep and waking can vary in several different ways. There is one sleep episode with one waking episode in most people, but some individuals have multiple sleep periods or multiple waking periods. The length of sleep is clearly affected to a major degree by age. With aging, the characteristics of sleep may change. Disturbance of nighttime sleep in the elderly has been reported by many sleep researchers and "napping" is frequent in this age group.

How sleep patterns change with environmental factors remains a fertile area of investigation. Studies of sleep in animals show the importance of biological rhythms which are highly responsive to light and dark conditions. While continuous darkness seems to have relatively little effect on established biological rhythms over a 24-hour period, the exposure to light tends to abolish these biological rhythms (See the section in Chapter 2 entitled, **Switching Out the Lights**)

Prolonged Wakefulness

Healthy individuals deprived of sleep suffer from a wide range of mental and physical disabilities. Extended deprivation of sleep for five days can make some individuals go berserk; and, at the very least, they can have major mood swings and even hallucinations. After a day or two of sleep deprivation, difficulty in focusing vision, nausea, memory lapses and delusions often occur. However, if the person is healthy, long-term personality changes or impaired performance do not persist after short periods of restful sleep which permit rapid recuperation.

Physical and Mental Impairment Due to Insomnia

Impairment in mental and physical activities due to prolonged wakefulness or sleep deprivation comes and goes in an unpredictable manner. In other words, these disabilities take the form of lapses of physical and mental abilities. Researchers have talked about the analogy between sleep deprivation and a "stuttering engine." This "engine" runs for a while, occasionally falters, sometimes stops and operates in "fits and starts". In brief, there is much variation among individuals in their response to sleep deprivation. Performance of physical or mental tasks in the presence of deprivation of sleep follows an interesting cycle itself. In the sleep deprived, their best physical or mental performance usually occurs in the evening and their poorest performance usually occurs in the early morning. The results of any stress in a sleep-deprived person are often magnified. A "short fuse" is found in the insomniac.

The time taken to recover from sleep deprivation by "recovery sleep" varies among individuals. However, it is generally noted that even after one night of high quality, recovery sleep there is often a rapid and dramatic reversal of physical and mental impairment caused by sleep deprivation. However, recovery is not instantaneous. Feelings of fatigue often persist for two or three days after prolonged periods of sleep deprivation and EEG recordings may not go back to normal for about 72 hours. Scientists have looked for drugs or chemicals that may accelerate recovery from sleep deprivation, but no clear, safe and effective "quick-fix" has been discovered to combat sleep deficits. Denying the body sleep is like borrowing money; it has to be paid back, often with a high interest rate!

Sleep is Affected by Lifestyle

Problems with sleep often have their roots in adverse lifestyle. Causes of poor sleep include unhealthy or poor timing of eating habits, lack of exercise, substance abuse, disordered daily routines and stress, often linked to anxiety.

Insomnia may be short-term or chronic (extended over a long period of time). One of the commonest causes of disturbed sleep patterns is traveling, especially if travel is through several time zones. A switch in time zones alters an individual's biological clock. Travelers may experience mild forms of insomnia due to changes in environment or even sleeping in an unfamiliar bed or bedroom.

Current estimates indicate that about 30 million Americans suffer from transient or short-term insomnia. While many of these people may overcome this problem by the use of natural ways to promote healthy sleep, many insomniacs jump to use drugs to help them sleep. Natural pathways to healthy sleep must be preferred. This approach is part of a "Sleep Naturally Plan" that is described in detail in this book. A combination of lifestyle change, behavior modification and natural adjuncts to healthy sleep are the bases of "the Plan."

Adjuncts to the first-line options of behavior modification include the use of natural, herbal, botanical and nutrient agents in dietary supplements (www.sleepnaturally.com or www.naturesbenefit.com). To achieve sleep in a natural way is an important part of a healthy lifestyle and it is known to contribute to health and well-being.

Sleep in the Elderly and the Young

The elderly are particularly susceptible to changes in their sleeping environment. For example, elderly people who have lived at home in a familiar environment may suffer major disorientation when their sleep surroundings are changed. This phenomenon is seen sometimes when elderly people are admitted to institutions or hospitals and, on occasion, severe episodes of nocturnal confusion may occur.

Sleep may seem to many people to be an acquired habit. For example, some children can only sleep while cuddling their favorite teddy bear. Thus, human traits such as rituals and minor obsessions are often important in sustaining normal sleep patterns. Like most habits, disruption of a familiar pattern of activities may disturb sleep.

Protracted Insomnia

More than 35 million Americans have chronic (long term) insomnia and in some cases it can be severe with associated physical and mental problems. Chronic insomniacs can become distraught by their inability to sleep. Some insomniacs report how they seek relief in watching TV or engaging in repetitive tasks (e.g. knitting, surfing the Internet, writing, etc.), but these millions of sleepless people invariably reach for medications to help themselves sleep, without exercising first-line natural ways to promote healthy sleep.

Degrees of Daytime Sleepiness

Sleepiness is subject to much subjective interpretation. There are people with apparently "sleepy personalities". The assessment of a degree of an individual's sleepiness has been made by simple "scales" or measures that can classify an individual's degree of sleepiness as mild, moderate or severe or worse. For general reference, a person who falls asleep while engaged in a conversation, driving a car or eating dinner must be considered to have a severe rating on a sleepiness scale.

The moderate type of "Rip van Winkle" is the person who falls asleep at work, during a long driving expedition or while engaged in interactions with family members. Moderate sleepiness must be considered to be present even if a man falls asleep while talking to his mother-in-law – this is not an excuse! Many of us fall into the rating of mild sleepiness when we dose while watching TV, attending lectures, riding in a car or reading this book. Sleepy persons rarely develop an objective opinion about their own degree of sleepiness. Such opinions are often more reliable from close social contacts. The ultimate form of sleepiness is called narcolepsy, where excessive daytime sleepiness occurs in association with altered mental and physical functions, disturbances of REM sleep and other specific sleep disturbances. Narcolepsy is surprisingly common. It affects about one in 150 of the population.

With all the sleeping aid devices and pills available in the market, one wonders why the number of insomniacs in America is increasing. The answer rests in the notion that few sleeping aids or devices work in a satisfactory or universal manner. Clearly, current initiatives to assist in healthy sleep possess many disadvantages and limitations. The "Sleep Naturally Plan" is a multi-pronged natural approach to restful sleep designed to make a difference to the widespread problem of insomnia.

Many Causes and Results of Insomnia

Failure of an individual to obtain healthy sleep has been the subject of numerous clinical and laboratory studies. These studies show that disordered sleep is due to many different and sometimes complex causes. Insomnia is a recurring "illness" for many people, but many people in America have adopted intentionally a nocturnal lifestyle.

Electronic games and surfing the Internet are a major factor in sleep deprivation in the young. Nocturnal teenagers become nocturnal adults and "practiced" lifestyle patterns can be quite difficult to change.

I have previously noted that the amount of sleep and its quality decline as people get older, but infants and toddlers often sleep for many hours. By the time a child turns 10 years old, sleeping time is reduced frequently to about 10 hours. Many adolescents and teenagers need at least 8 hours of sleep, but recent population studies show that many may only sleep for 6 or 7 hours, or less. The multimedia revolution has played a major role in the development of the "teenage night owl."

The Eight-Hour Sleep

Eight-hour sleep is often proposed as the ideal duration of sleeping time. I stress that 8 hours cannot be regarded as a gospel statement; and it is certainly not a magic number. However, it is the number of hours that many experts suggest as optimal so that the body can experience all normal five phases of sleep. Good quality sleep is characterized by progression through the normal multiple stages which add up to complete physical and mental rest. The body needs to complete these stages of sleep to get a complete physical rest (early sleep) and to achieve control over memory, learning and mood (later sleep). The later stages of sleep are required for the brain to retain information for the learning process. Reductions in sleep can result in irritability, distractedness, tiredness, absent-mindedness and poor cognitive function. Sleep deprived individuals are slow to react to things around them.

There is a condition known as "subjective insomnia" which is often associated with anxiety and/or variable degrees of depression. While people with subjective insomnia are not necessarily shortchanged on the duration of their sleep, their sleep is often of poor quality. The person with subjective insomnia has sleep that can be easily disrupted. Individuals with subjective insomnia may wake up with a hangover and a lack of sensation of refreshment as a consequence of sleeping. However, their complaints of "lack of sleep" are perceived rather than experienced.

Substituting Cavalier Approaches to Sleep

Some people with insomnia have developed a cavalier attitude towards the use of drugs to help them sleep. Physicians and sleep experts have warned sleep-deprived individuals against the dangers of self-medication with hypnotic drugs, but the chronic insomniac may be desperate enough to try almost anything to help them sleep. While new sleeping drugs have appeared in the market with proclaimed advantages of a shorter duration of action, these shorter-acting medications can cause drug dependency and hangover. The attitude of some insomniacs to use "whatever works" must be challenged as alternative medicine presents holistic, simpler and safe approaches to natural sleep with selected herbs and nutritional factors (www.sleepnaturally.com).

Drugs, such as benzodiazepines and antihistamines, are frequently used by people with disordered sleep, but side effects from prolonged use of these drugs are more common than reports may suggest. Dietary supplements containing natural substances that provide nutritional support for healthy sleep are gaining increasing acceptance as alternatives to sleeping drugs (see Chapter 6 and www.sleepnaturally.com). Practitioners of alternative medicine are using natural sleeping aids in dietary supplements increasingly to switch away from drug use (see Chapter 6, www.sleepnaturally.com).

Invoking Positive Lifestyle

The change from an adverse to a healthy lifestyle is the most appropriate way to "jumpstart" the effective management of sleep disorders. This approach is healthy and safe. Many simple interventions may promote sleep. Nutritional approaches that are as fundamental as the drinking of a glass of warm milk at night may be effective for some people. While such advice sounds like an "old wives' cure," milk contains amino acids, which are known to have a calming effect on the central nervous system.

Close attention to several specific aspects of lifestyle can promote healthy sleep. Exercise has panacea health benefits, but strenuous exercise prior to retiring at night can actually induce arousal and interfere with sleep. The promotion of psychological well-being and good eating patterns also help sleep. Simple interventions, such as mental imagery or meditation, are quite valuable adjuncts (see Chapter 5). For the committed person, yoga has real value in resetting biological clocks and assisting sleep.

Sleep is Part of a Healthy Lifestyle

Experts underscore the value of making good sleep habits an integral part of a healthy lifestyle. Preparations for bedtime must begin with activity that calms the body. Some activities such as light stretching exercises, meditation or prayer, reading a book or watching TV, can help the body to wind down prior to sleep. To involve the "would-be sleeper" in discussions about conflicts or problems should be excluded from bedroom chatter. Such discussions serve only to introduce anxiety and tension before sleep. Taking work into the bedroom is a common pathway to insomnia. The bedroom is a sanctuary for rest and relaxation and the bed must be reserved as a platform for comfort, sleep and intimacy. Restful sleep is a fundamental domain of a healthy lifestyle.

Why We Sleep?

Sleep finds meaning for many people in the concepts of restoration and recovery of the body. Humankind must engage in energy conservation. While these concepts are imprinted in many people's minds, the reason we sleep remains poorly understood. I am inclined to believe that sleep is not to be considered a time of body inactivity. In fact, certain periods of sleep, e.g. rapid eye movement sleep (REM), are associated with much active body function. Sleep can be considered a form of modified consciousness.

I believe that sleep needs may be related to the need for "electric circuits" created by chemical reactions to rebalance themselves. The chemistry of life may be like a battery, in simplistic terms, and it requires a period of recharging. In this context of recharging, I refer mainly to electrical activities in cells or their membranes, e.g. proton pumps.

Most people find the need to sleep as a means of recovering lost energy or recuperating from day-to-day activity. During sleep, the brain goes into a temporary phase of relaxation, but it also goes into phases of great excitations. It is clear that sleep is not for rest alone. Simple sleep may be an adequate respite for muscles, bones, joints and some body organs, but the complexities of sleep functions are necessary to support the central nervous system. The brain must experience sleep in order to learn and engage in ordered, higher mental activity. Research has shown a clear connection between sleep and learning. Furthermore, sleep deprivation can cause much suffering from mood disturbance.

Lessons from Animals

Like animals, humans do not rest in the face of danger. Humankind's cultural evolution has brought with it a sense of security. In contrast, lower animals have their own peculiar and varied needs for sleep habitats and habitats of sleep. Many animals of prey hide during sleep and only rest with the security of self-preservation. This habitat prevents the attraction of predators. It is notable that successful predators may sleep openly without the same fears of danger. A pride of lions is willing to bask in the open, whereas animals of prey dig holes underground or sleep inside caves and tunnels.

Major differences in sleeping habits are observed among different animal species. While a giraffe sleeps about 2 hours, baboons sleep usually more than 9 hours and bats up to 20 hours! There are several theories to explain these differences in sleep duration. Experts in animal behavior proposed one theory: they believe that the different sleep patterns are related to whether or not an animal is common prey or a predator. These hypotheses could be extended to different behavioral attributes among humans. While the concept of predator and prey is not readily applied to humans, one could substitute the idea of assertive and passive behavior. Certainly, one expects the more passive individual to have fewer problems with sleep, but this is not always the case. Outward displays of passivity in humans may hide inner aggression and vice versa?

In brief, it is suggested that prey animals have short periods of sleep for reasons of self preservation. The vulnerable animal lives with the fear of being attacked and this dictates extended periods of sleeplessness. The human with anxieties or fears may share extended periods of sleeplessness, just like a frightened animal. Scared animals, like anxious humans, are not able to sleep when they sense danger or discomfort lurking in their surroundings. Thus, the suitability of the environment in which one sleeps is "all important."

Is Napping Healthy?

"Napping" defies definition and it has different connotations in different ethnic groups. Some individuals believe in the refreshing nature of "power napping", where periods of sleep, no longer than 30 minutes, are alleged to be refreshing. Power napping is not known to be healthy and it cannot be considered a substitute for good sleep. In Hispanic communities, napping is extended to the notion of "the siesta". The effect of napping on nocturnal sleeplessness produces mixed results. Daytime napping, in any form, is not recommended for the insomniac or the elderly, as it can detract from nighttime sleep.

Sleeping Rituals

The idea of promoting comfort, security and well-being to invite sleep is neither novel nor new, but it can be quite effective. Various cultures have observed bedtime rituals from ancient times. The hum of a lullaby, a relaxing shower, reading a book or changing into comfortable clothes are simple acts that are sometimes overlooked by the poor sleeper. These rituals are traditionally identified with preparations for bedtime. However, sleep can be elusive to individuals with unhealthy rituals. Substance abuse is the exact antithesis of sleep; and the chemicals in alcoholic beverages, cigarettes, sedatives or prescription drugs are capable of interfering with the normal functions of the brain that control sleep.

Revisiting Gender Differences in Sleep Patterns

I have noted earlier that women have more apparent problems than men in getting a good night's sleep. The records of the National Sleep Foundation show that up to 60% of all women between the ages of 30 and 60 years have trouble sleeping. Sleep problems in women occur with a frequency in the population similar to the status of being overweight (60% of the population). However, much more emphasis is placed on weight control than sleep balance when it comes to health. One cannot "touch or feel" sleep problems, but one can readily notice bulging waistlines. An important consideration is that both obesity and poor sleep are major health risks; and, often, they go "hand-in-hand."

Population studies indicate that twice as many women than men suffer attacks of sleepiness during the day. Furthermore, about 25% of all women over the age of 30 have difficulty in falling asleep or staying asleep on a regular basis. The reasons for the preponderance in "simple" sleep problems in women are unclear, but overt alteration in hormonal balances in women cause sleep disorders, e.g. PMS and menopause.

Lack of Sleep Causes Premature Aging

Who would think that good sleep is an important anti-aging tactic? Sleep deprivation over a prolonged period of time affects adversely the function of all body organs. One mechanism whereby lack of sleep wreaks havoc with several body structures and functions is through its effects on body hormones and changes in the metabolism of the body (the chemistry of life).

Research studies on a variety of blood hormones show major changes in hormonal imbalances in sleep-deprived young adults. Scientists have found that the pattern of blood hormones in young people who slept only four hours per night for one week changed to a body hormone profile similar to that most often found in older people. Further studies have shown that the sleep-deprived volunteers became resistant to the actions of the master hormone "insulin." This type of hormonal disturbance is found in Syndrome X, where one finds hypertension, high blood cholesterol and obesity linked by the occurrence of "resistance to the hormone insulin." Syndrome X affects up to 70 million Americans. Syndrome X is emerging as America's number one public health initiative (www.combatsyndromex.com) and it seems to be related, in part, to sleep deprivation.

Of particular note in these research studies of blood hormones was falling levels of growth hormone with sleep deprivation. Growth hormone typically falls in the blood with advancing years. Moreover, researchers have shown declines in muscle tissue (loss of muscle mass) and impairments in body immunity in the subjects who restricted their sleep.

These studies present some compelling evidence to view sleep deprivation as a factor that contributes to premature aging. A logical conclusion to these studies is that good sleep may be a key to anti-aging initiatives. One may now understand why the prince who kissed the sleeping princess was rewarded by her youthful attributes.

Chapter Summary

There are many factors that control the duration and quality of sleep. Healthy sleep is an absolute prerequisite for general well-being. This chapter summarizes some of the many issues that place sleep into its correct health perspective. The study of sleep and the management of sleep disorders have come to the forefront of medical science in the past decade. This renaissance of interest in sleep has occurred as a consequence of many research studies that show the negative health and social outcomes of poor sleep.

As we explore current information on the significance of sleep for general well-being, a rational series of proposals emerge as first-line options to help the "poor sleeper." The notion that America may be able to "Sleep Naturally," using natural ways to healthy sleep, forms part of important public health initiatives for this new millennium.

Chapter 2:

SLEEPING, DREAMING AND BIOLOGICAL CLOCKS

Historical Perspectives on Sleep

Sleep has fascinated people from time immemorial. Early written accounts of sleep gave the impression that observers thought that sleeping people looked like they were stricken with paralysis. Reports of people seeing self-created images during sleep led to the study of dreams. At the turn of the 20th century, behavioral scientists started to interpret the act of dreaming which is seen as one of life's great mysteries, even today.

Early scientific hypotheses to explain sleep disorders can be traced to the start of the 19th century. One such theory to explain sleep disturbance was that lack of sleep was caused by the brain being excessively congested with blood. These early notions were replaced by ideas that the brain accumulated toxic substances during periods of wakefulness and these toxic substances were discharged during sleep. The elimination of toxins by sleep was believed to result in "body regeneration" following periods of rest. This theory has been reactivated in modern times by describing links between the bacterial populations of the colon and sleep.

Other theories likened sleep to an "on-and-off reflex condition," somewhat similar to an electric switch. While it was once believed that sleep was a condition of inactivity, this notion was replaced by the new concepts of the presence of an active brain within a periodically motionless body. Many scientists have commented on the rhythms of sleep and wakefulness by night and day. Even these days, correlations between darkness and sleep or light and wakefulness are unclear.

Sleep Deprivation Can Have Tragic Consequences

During times of public upheaval or conflict, the sleep of a nation can be disturbed. Valuable information about the body functions of sleep comes from unusual sources. Scientists and sociologists can learn much from the consequences of sleep deprivation during times of war. Nowhere is this problem more apparent than in recent conflicts between Western and Middle Eastern nations. More than a decade ago, the media highlighted a tragic event where an incident of "friendly fire" during the Gulf War of 1990 resulted in the tragic death of several people.

This incident of "friendly fire" in the 1990 Gulf War conflict involved an American Marine who accidentally shot and killed his fellow soldiers. At the time of the incident, the reasons for its occurrence were not clear. Ten years later, investigations led to the conclusion that this apparent senseless human act occurred as a consequence of lack of sleep experienced by the American Marine in question. Sleep experts in the military say that in a day's cycle of 24 hours, war-weary soldiers may only get an average of three to five hours of sleep. The loss of human lives is an extreme example of the catastrophic consequences of sleep deprivation.

Brain Functions and Sleep

In 1809, Luigi Rolando, an Italian neuroscientist, discovered alterations in brain electrical functions with different sleep patterns. By stimulating the brain with electricity, this scientist observed differences in sleep patterns. This paved the way for many succeeding experiments that clearly linked sleep patterns with changing functions of the central nervous system.

Further information about sleep came from the unusual source of botanical science. Botanists of the 19th century observed periodic activity in plants, such as the opening and closing of flowers. This movement in plants was likened to sleep and waking patterns in humans. The famous Swedish botanist, Carolus Linnaeus, studied thousands of plants which led to his discoveries of the effect of the environment on the movement of plants. These early observations are incorporated into modern concepts of the orchestration and harmony of life forms in our biosphere. Over the years, the rhythm of life has become apparent. Life events in plants and animals are viewed as parallels to human life events.

The Sleeping Eyes Tell a Story: Rapid Eye Movement Sleep (REM)

Eye movements during sleep were noted by William Griesinger in 1868, but it was not until 1953 when rapid eye movement (REM) during sleep became placed in its impartial perspective. At this time, REM were studied in detail and linked to the current understanding of sleeping and dreaming. The use of the electroencephalogram (EEG) to monitor brain waves during sleep was introduced in 1929. The EEG permitted the recording of electrical activity in the brain, which led to a refinement of the theories behind REM sleep. Using the EEG in 1937, a group of scientists observed regular sleep cycles and classified them into several stages. These different stages of sleep occur with variable duration and timing in the healthy individual.

Sleep Is an Active State

A breakthrough came in 1953 with the validation and study of the rapid eye movement phase (REM) of sleep. Studies by Nathaniel Kleitman and his student Eugene Aserinsky started to reject the notion that sleep was a condition of inactivity. Their studies found sleep to be an "active state." Bursts of brain activity during REM sleep supported their emerging theories. The researchers also recorded muscle activity, blood pressure and heart palpitations during sleep. Part of the Kleitman-Aserinsky experiments was to wake up subjects during REM sleep, and have the subjects recall their dreams. For these landmark studies, Kleitman earned the title of "Father of American Sleep Research."

Kleitman's studies impacted current understanding of sleep and wakefulness with the focus on the presence of the "Circadian Rhythm." The Circadian Rhythm is essentially a cycle of sleep and wakefulness linked with many changes in body function. In a classic research paper by Kleitman entitled "Sleep and Wakefulness," it was proposed that a combination of factors were likely to induce sleep. These factors included "tiring" of the central nervous system and the absence of stimulation in the environment. These simplistic notions have been elaborated in their complexities by modern research.

Dreaming: Sigmund Freud Hits the Mark

Dreaming became a fascinating area of research in the late Victorian era. The work entitled, "The Interpretation of Dreams," was Sigmund Freud's original thesis on dreams as a reflection of the human persona. Freud's book was published in 1899 and it provided some insights into dreaming that were very controversial during his time, but his work gained acceptance after his death in 1939. Freud was best known as the "Father of Psychoanalysis" and in his book on dream analyses, Freud proposed several concepts about dreaming, but his preoccupation with sex led to him being labeled as a "pervert" by the conservative society of his era.

Sigmund Freud noted that dreams fade away in the morning and many who experienced them may not entirely recall all the details after their awakening. Some people completely forget their dreams, whereas others seem to recall them with all their colorful details. Freud believed that dreams were a fulfillment of wishes that an individual had that were stored beneath their conscious level. In other words, these "subconscious wishes" were expressed in dreams and represented what a person may want to attain during wakeful periods.

Sigmund Freud attempted to distinguish two main types of dreaming. On the one hand, he described the idea of "latent dreams" which were essentially personal desires, whereas on the other hand, Freud described "manifest dreams." Manifest dreams are typified by the way in which the dreamer directly participates in the events of the dream. People are not often aware they are dreaming. With dreaming, the body often experiences rapid eye movement (REM), twitching and other forms of body responses that are triggered by brain activity, in complex and still poorly understood ways.

The Significance of Dreams

Most people "cast off" their experiences during dreaming. From ancient times, dreams have been viewed as anything ranging from unimportant fantasies to serious omens of events to come. A large amount of material about dreaming has been synthesized by psychologists and other scientists, but the significance of dreams remains quite debatable. Varying durations and types of dreams come to all people at one or other times in their life, but the occurrence of dreams and their apparent meaning remains underexplored.

The Bible contains rich accounts of the significance of dreams; and there are many books written on dream contents and their potential significance. I tend to agree with the common suggestion that dreams are a type of "sleep thought" and they are a reflection of daily experiences. Table 4 gives some examples of the content of dreams and their significance. Whether or not there is any substance to the interpretation of dream content is quite contentious.

The Origin of Dreams

Scientists have toiled with their understanding of what causes an individual to dream. It is suggested that there are "reflex actions" in the brain that occur during sleep. These reflex actions are affected by the distortion of daily events or perceptions. It may be that same daily events are so strongly imprinted on a person's mind that they become the focus of memory recall during dreaming. Some dreams appear to be composed of lucid events, but some are merely a jumble of confusing sights and sounds. These "jumbled dreams" often have physical causes such as gastrointestinal upset, emotional disturbances and other physical or psychological causes. The jumbled dream may be a sign of a "body not at ease with itself."

Dream Experience	**Possible Meaning**
A bag or baggage	Believed to be a sign of better times ahead, especially if the bag appears heavy
A book or books	Generally thought to be a good sign, suggesting future happiness
Airplane or airplanes	Signifies potential fortune when flying, but if crashing may indicate a business failure
A dead body, corpse	Regarded as a potential omen of separation from friends or loved ones as a consequence of one's own fault
The devil	Generally considered a bad dream which must involve long struggles in the future
A juggler	A sign of advancement in one's position in life that may become within a person's grasp. Considered an opportunity that should be taken without hesitation
Rain	Perhaps a legacy or a present.

Table 4 : Some examples of the potential meaning of the content of some dreams. There are books that describe long lists of dream content or objects within dreams that are supposed to have specific meaning. The above examples were modified from the book, entitled "Dreams and Omens", Foulsham's "New" Popular Handbook, Ward J, W. Foulsham and Co. Ltd., London, UK, circa 1950.

Digestive Upset and Sleep Disturbance

In the clinical practice of gastroenterology, I have found many people with nighttime digestive disturbances who complain of "jumbled dreams." A particularly common clinical combination is the occurrence of jumbled dreams in the presence of nocturnal heartburn. Sometimes, these patients with heartburn (or upper abdominal discomfort) had eaten late in the evening and they had been often drinking alcohol. Certainly, alcohol and other drugs can precipitate "jumbled" patterns of dreaming. Among the many books written on sleep disturbance, authors have rarely commented on the common relationship between digestive upset and sleep deprivation.

It is known that balanced digestive function promotes healthy sleep. Theories exist about the healthy bacterial environment of the colon (bowel) and the occurrence of restful sleep. Certainly, during sleep the digesta (contents of the colon) play a role in balancing general body functions. One important "balancing function" is the ability of friendly bacteria in the bowel to prime immune function. At night, the normal "by-products" of friendly types of bacteria in the bowel may cause the release of "body messenger" chemicals (interleukins) that help to induce sleep. Thus, the contents of the bowel are "talking" indirectly to the brain. The control of digestive upset is an important but often overlooked factor in many people with sleeplessness (Holt S, Natural Ways to Digestive Health, M. Evans Publishers, NY, NY, 2000).

There are natural ways to help control upper digestive function, including the alteration of the secretion of acid by the stomach. Suppression of stomach acid is a key initiative in dealing with common upper digestive discomforts. Reduction in acid secretion or neutralization of stomach acid is most often achieved by drugs, but natural products have become available that have both immediate neutralizing ability and powerful antioxidant components that may suppress the secretion of stomach acid (Zanasec™, www.zanasec.com). In addition to natural or drug-induced attempts to control acid secretion, correct posture during sleep is very important. The adoption of a semi-upright position at night helps to control the "backwash of acid" from the stomach into the esophagus (gastroesophageal reflux). This backwash of acid causes heartburn and other unpleasant digestive symptoms.

The backwash of acid is called "acid reflux"; and it may be part of a condition called gastroesophageal reflux disease (GERD). Sleeping with extra pillows placed in careful positions or "propping the head of the bed" on books or bricks can be quite effective in stopping acid reflux (backwash of acid from stomach to gullet or esophagus). Sometimes, the reflux of gastric acid into the esophagus can result in choking sensations or even serious respiratory disorders during sleep. There are some people with acid reflux who wake up with a sore throat due to acid irritation at the back of their throat; and sometimes, individuals may wake up with hoarseness as a consequence of the irritation of the vocal chords by refluxed acid. These symptoms require medical attention and, if left untreated, this severity of acid reflux can result in complications of GERD.

Sleep Has a Chemical Basis

Many "chemicals" have an impact on sleep. French scientists Rene Legendre and Henri Pieron suggested the presence of a "hypnotoxin," a body chemical present in sleep-deprived dogs. When this crude "hypnotoxin" was injected into dogs with normal sleep patterns, this would make them sleep. The suggestion of the presence of sleep-inducing chemicals within the body was contradicted by the celebrated Russian physiologist Ivan Pavlov of the "Pavlovian Classical Conditioning Theory." However, modern research in dogs with "narcolepsy" (falling asleep at the drop of a hat) may support the idea of specific "sleep hormones." These days, scientists have much information on the complex biochemical control of sleep (see Chapters 5, 6 and 7).

Sleep and a Wide Variety of Behaviors

In the 19th and 20th centuries, sleep was analyzed by all branches of medical science, including botany and pharmacology. The idea that sleep is not a state of paralysis has gathered a wide following. Over the past century, scientists have refined their hypotheses about sleep control and found that as the body lies immobile in sleep, major body organs all function in synchronicity with one another. In sleep, eyelids flicker, toes quiver, lungs heave, and heart rate and blood pressure soar and fall. The dynamics experienced by a sleeping body are quite dramatic and they can include sleepwalking in some children and a consistent occurrence of penile erections in young healthy men, or vaginal lubrication in women. While some slumbering people mumble in their sleep, others may become infrequently violent. All of these behaviors are a major focus of modern research.

The Biological Clock Ticks

In the 1950s, the concept of a "biological clock" was put forward by Gustav Kramer and Klaus Hoffman. These proposals "picked up" on earlier theories about the analogies of plant movements and human sleep, such as the opening and folding of leaves and petals at certain hours of the day. Kramer and Hoffman observed the patterns of migration in birds and concluded their flight was determined by the sunshine and time zones. These types of observations were made by many scientists and formed the basis of the ideas that orchestration existed between living matter and the biosphere (earth and universe). The rhythm and harmony of life are still underestimated in their importance in modern medicine.

The idea of the presence of a "biological clock" caught on in humans in the past century. This notion of a "built-in body clock" was bolstered by a series of experiments in the 1960s and 1970s which advanced theories by studying the influence of light and dark in sleep patterns. In these experiments, human subjects were kept underground for a period of time and insulated from normal environmental influences. Their sleep-wake cycles were measured. Researchers who plotted aspects of "biological clocks" found them to be slightly longer than a regular 24-hour period.

The "biological clock" or the Circadian Rhythm became an acceptable concept in modern medicine after scientists discovered activity of specific parts of the brain linked to the biological clock. This activity involved the function of a part of the brain called the suprachiasmatic nuclei (SCN). This location in the brain is active on both sides of the hypothalamus during a regular sleep-wake cycle. Like a "bandleader," this portion of the brain appears to play a major role in coordinating sleep and wakefulness in the same way that musical harmonies are created.

Switching Out the Lights

In a fascinating book written by T.S. Wiley and Bent Formby ("Lights Out," Simon and Schuster Inc, NY, 2000), the role of artificial light in the promotion of sleep deprivation is reviewed in explicit detail. This book is very hard to read, but it is worth the investment of time, in order to unravel its messages. Wiley and Formby interpret information obtained from research studies performed largely at the National Institutes of Health (NIH) and the National Institute of Mental Health (NIMH) in Washington DC. The authors refer to some of their conclusions in a cute manner by referring to this government-sponsored research as the "secret of NIMH", referring specifically to the National Institute of Mental Health (NIMH). The book by Wiley and Formby suffers from a series of "catchy" subheadings which do not always reflect the content of the sections to which they apply. In common with many other contemporary researchers, Wiley and Formby provide a hypothesis that America is becoming increasingly unwell as a consequence of sleep deprivation.

The authors of "Lights Out" reached some puzzling and contrarian conclusions where they even deny the benefits of strenuous exercise and reactivate some nonsensical notions that calories may not count when it comes to weight control. Although these authors raise very challenging concepts, they have engaged in the utmost "lateral thinking" – an act worthy of much praise. Drawing upon knowledge about the way the universe functions in harmony (a modified Gaia hypothesis) and the way lifestyles once were, prior to the introduction of artificial light (the light bulb), the authors indicate that modern humankind is reacting against its own innate characteristics.

In other words, the authors of "Lights Out" present an argument that the balance of nature, with alternating periods of light and dark (day and night), is imprinted in our normal body physiology (body functions). Invoking standard and accepted consequences of biological rhythms, it is apparent that changes in body chemistry, such as hormone secretions, occur in synchronicity (in sync) from day to day. These proposals are part of the established concepts of the "harmony of life" (an aphorism of the cruel vivisectionist Claude Bernard).

Modern Society Lives with Deceptive Daylight

The chemistry of life is highly dependent upon balanced secretions of hormones and chemicals which cause the transmission of nervous impulses in the central nervous system. This balanced body chemistry forms the basis of normal mental and physical functioning. It has been proposed by T.S. Wiley and B. Formby that modern civilizations have relied heavily upon artificial light to extend their days into the night. In simple terms, it is suggested that these extended periods of artificial light deceive the body. This deception gives the body the impression that it is living in a perpetual state of daylight or summer.

Drawing upon experiences from animals that hibernate, this line of reasoning suggests that the body lives with the erroneous perception that summer is constant. "Constant summer" means "constant stress" upon the body. The analogy is that during the summer, animals engage in "fattening themselves up" and other stressful activity that prepares them for a period of hibernation or winter. In the wintertime, animal activity is characteristically restricted and food supply is scarce.

It has been proposed that excessive light exposure (constant daylight or summer) makes the body store fat and prepare itself for the slowing down of its chemistry to help prepare to sustain itself through months of hibernation or restricted activities of winter. According to Wiley and Formby, this preparation for "winter" in animals is not a good thing and it is not relevant or healthy for modern humankind. The "artificial summer" created by prolonged exposures to "artificial lights" is not followed by phases of "classic winter."

Lack of Sleep and Disease Profiles

Strange as it may seem to some, the book by Wiley and Formby talks about getting at least 9 hours of sleep a night and claims that this act will result in: weight loss, reduction in craving for carbohydrate, eradication of depression or other mental illnesses, lowering of blood pressure, stress reduction, reversal of Type 2 maturity onset diabetes, reductions in the risk of heart disease and even the prevention of cancer. These are bold claims, but they may not be entirely without foundation.

I find the controversial conclusions of Wiley and Formby particularly interesting and I am impressed with some of the reasoning behind sleep deprivation and the biochemistry of weight gain or the modern evolution of Syndrome X (obesity, high blood pressure and high blood cholesterol linked by insulin resistance). We have learned that healthy sleep-deprived individuals develop insulin resistance (See Chapter 1); and insulin resistance is a pivotal factor in the cause of the metabolic Syndrome X.

Insulin is one of the many hormones that are affected by sleep deprivation. Others include growth hormone, melatonin, cortisol, glucagon, etc. Sleep deprivation seems to promote insulin resistance and modern studies confirm this. Perhaps a good night's sleep must be part of the combat against Syndrome X (Holt S, "Combat Syndrome X, Y and Z...", Wellness Publishing, Newark, NJ, 2002, and Holt S and Wright J, "Syndrome X Nutritional Factors," Wellness Publishing, Newark, NJ, 2003 www.combatsyndromex.com).

Too Much Sleep Can Be Unhealthy?

Clearly, there is no consensus on a healthy duration of sleep for everyone; and nor could there be given the different sleep requirements of different people of different ages. A recent study found that individuals who sleep 8 hours or more are prone to increased death rates than those who sleep 6 to 7 hours. The findings concluded that individuals who sleep 8 hours are 12% more likely to die within six years than those sleeping 7 or even 5 hours a night. For example, women who snooze 9 to 11 hours appear to be more prone to heart disease than those who sustain 8 hours or less of sleep.

According to this recent study, individuals who sleep an average of 6.5 hours a night may be reassured that this is a "safe" amount of sleep. The researchers concluded that from a health standpoint, there is no reason to sleep longer. While some research studies support these conclusions, others tell a different story. I reiterate that there is no consensus opinion on the optimal time for health and some studies imply that longer sleep times can be healthy.

Biorhythms

Astrologers and behavioral scientists are developing hypotheses which make their disciplines move together. For more than a millennium, evidence has existed that healers and patients have tried to take account of physical or mental cycles in their day-to-day life. At the start of the 20th century, Dr. Wilhelm Fleiss investigated and promoted the notions that there were "Physical Cycles" in humankind that governed events such as birth, death and the development of disease.

Added to the notion of the presence of a "Physical Cycle" was the proposal that there was an "Emotional Cycle." Dr. Fleiss was a close colleague of Dr. Sigmund Freud and Freud supported Fleiss' concepts of biological rhythms. Freud's preoccupation with sex resulted in disagreements between these noble gentlemen. In fact, Sigmund Freud proposed that dream analysis had confirmed the existence of an "Emotional Cycle" or emotional biorhythm. The arguments between Drs. Freud and Fleiss were fueled by Dr. Hermann Swoboda, who received awards for work on biorhythms.

Other distinguished scientists proposed the presence of an "Intellectual Cycle." The presence of an Intellectual Cycle was used to explain why an individual's intellectual performance would vary from day to day or week to week. There is some evidence that Intellectual Cycles do exist and such cycles may be related to differences in hormone secretions by the body or other changes in body chemistry.

It is proposed by experts in biorhythms that there are three natural and regular cycles, occurring in men and women (physical, emotional and intellectual). An awareness of the presence and status of certain characteristics of biorhythm may assist some people in regulating the quality of their life and improving well-being. There is no doubt that sleep cycles are part of biorhythms and disturbed sleep may disturb the biorhythms. Conventional medicine has taken relatively little notice of the presence of biorhythm, perhaps because this area of science seems to be a strange mix of hypotheses, scientific observations and speculation.

It is clear that the human body handles events in a different manner, depending upon Circadian Rhythm or other biorhythms. Differences have been noted in the response to medications at different times during the day or night and moods can change dramatically at different times of the year. There are well described diseases that are linked to biological rhythms that are disturbed by environmental factors. A classic example is "Seasonal Affective Disorder" where exposure to excessive darkness or lack of light may contribute to depression and other mood disorders. In simple terms, humankind is not always "marching to the regular beat" of Nature and help may be required to place biological rhythms "back on track," so that they function with optimal synchronicity.

Solid Advice on Simple Approaches to Sleep

At this point in this book, I have reviewed a number of issues related to the understanding of sleep deprivation and simple facts about healthy sleep. It is prudent to define some simple measures that can promote healthy sleep without any recourse to medical interventions. Table 5 reviews simple measures that play a role in encouraging restful sleep.

- Assess your sleep duration and quality. Make a sleep journal, ask your sleeping partner about your sleep habits.
- Regularity in sleeping and waking patterns is important to set the stage for regular sleep cycles. Attempts to awaken and go to bed at similar times everyday are beneficial. Regimentation of sleep is a valuable activity.
- An individual who really cannot sleep should not spend long times lying in bed. On occasion, this person may be best advised to engage in activity.
- Daytime "napping" is an arch enemy of restful nocturnal sleep, especially in the elderly.
- Individuals should avoid dietary substances containing stimulants, such as caffeine and alcohol at night.
- Meditation and relaxation with some time to examine the events of the day is valuable in many insomniacs who cannot deal with "the worry of the day". The time for worrying is in the morning. If necessary, people can plan "daytime worrying sessions."
- A bed is for sleep and sex, not for work, worrying or eating.
- Pay good attention to the bedroom environment. Encourage partners to get help with their snoring. Otherwise, partners can be encouraged to sleep elsewhere, but this is not popular advice.
- If eating is planned in the two hours preceding bedtime then food choices must be appropriate, e.g. milk and light healthy snacks.
- Regular exercise helps sleep, but late night exercising must be abandoned.

- A new bed, good pillows all help.
- Individuals are advised not to wrestle with their inability to sleep.
- Pamper yourself before sleep.
- Develop bedtime rituals.
- Consider natural sleep aids, not drugs, as a first-line option (www.sleep-naturally.com).
- Consider a consultation with a sleep expert if you have long-standing problems or indications of a sleep disorder, such as sleepwalking or sleep apnea.

Table 5: Simple advice to help people sleep.

Chapter Summary

The farther back one looks at sleep science, the farther forward one can go (a modification of a Winston Churchill aphorism). We live in a universe characterized by a harmony of life. Sleep has a very important historical perspective that illustrates its importance for the maintenance of health and wellness. There are many facets to sleep which remain underexplored.

When persons develop a poor relationship with their own sleep patterns, they can suffer greatly. Any complementary approaches to improve sleep quality and duration for the millions of sleepless Americans must be welcomed. As we examine the science of sleep, behavioral changes required to induce healthy sleep become increasingly apparent and the use of natural agents to promote sleep starts to emerge with a well-defined role.

Chapter 3:
THE SCIENCE OF SLEEP

Ignoring Sleep Problems

The last decade has witnessed increasing medical interest in sleep disorders. In recent times, there have been several milestones in the reporting of the negative health consequences of sleep deprivation. The extent of sleep disorders was highlighted in the early 1990s in a report of the National Commission on Sleep Disorders Research which was published by the U.S. Department of Health and Human Services. More than a decade ago, 40 million U.S. citizens had problems with sleeplessness and its daytime consequences. These days, the numbers are revised upward to almost 100 million Americans.

Despite the common nature of sleep disorders, the reports by the Sleep Disorders Commission implied that many affected people did not seek medical advice for sleeplessness. Perhaps, these people did not consider their sleep problems to be serious enough to merit attention by physicians. While insomnia is the most common form of reported sleep disorder, there are more than 70 other types of sleep disturbances that have been identified in clinical research. The numerous abnormalities of sleep and wake patterns are caused by many factors.

Understanding Circadian Rhythms

The Circadian Rhythm is like a body clock that sets patterns of sleep and wakefulness. This rhythm dictates when the body should get its sleep or awaken. Modern lifestyles often work against the regularity of Circadian Rhythms. There are at least a couple of broad controlling mechanisms that operate the Circadian Rhythm. The first has been called a homeostatic mechanism. Homeostasis is really a state of balance in the body and it refers to the existence of a balance between sleep and wakefulness. Researchers have analyzed many factors that establish sleep tendencies over a period of about 24 hours. These factors are believed to be part of what has been called the "Circadian Oscillator."

Oscillators are responsible for changing a number of body functions. In fact, the word oscillate means to swing backwards and forwards with a steady but uninterrupted rhythm. Circadian Oscillators allow the body to make changes in its functions without alternations to extremes. This activity occurs in a defined period of time. Certainly, the Circadian Oscillator plays a major role in changing body temperatures, body hormone levels and chemicals involved in nerve transmissions throughout the central nervous system. While the actual names of the major controls of Circadian Rhythm are unimportant, it must be recognized that Circadian Oscillators and Homeostatic Mechanisms function in complete harmony in the normal individual and they are ultimately responsible for normal sleep cycles.

In other words, the Circadian Rhythm has been pre-set in many people to respond to certain times of the day. Lifestyle or environmental factors that disturb Circadian Rhythm are obvious causes of sleep disturbance. For example, shift workers who work at night and sleep by day are artificially reversing their "body clocks" and clearly altering their Circadian Rhythms. Furthermore, if these shift workers change from night to daytime shifts, they can make a "royal mess" of their biological clocks. In fact, several studies of shift workers have shown how disturbed "biological clocks" result in accidents or contribute to disease, with occasional tragic loss of lives.

The Role of Light in Sleep Cycles

While I have simplified explanations about the mechanisms that control sleep and wakefulness, one should recognize the response of biological clocks to light intensity. Generally speaking, the internal clock revolves around the presence or absence of light. When there is bright light the body often awakens. The human body has clever ways of detecting the light. In fact, the presence of light-sensitive receptors in many body tissues, apart from the eyes, has been proposed.

There is no doubt that the energy provided from light is a common basis for all life forms on the planet Earth, and perhaps other planets.

The most important effects of cycles of body exposure to light and dark include hormonal changes, release of chemicals that transmit nerve impulses and normal function of the immune system. Some experiments suggest that even focusing a strong beam of "pin point" light on the skin, when an individual is in a dark room, may alter sleep patterns.

In summary, there are five principal stages of sleep which can be associated with many mind and body events:

Presleep wake (sleep latency period): blinking of the eyes, limb movements and moderate tone in skeletal muscles

- Stage 1: slow rolling eye movements and sudden limb jerks may occur
- Stage 2: eye movements become infrequent or absent; muscle tone is reduced
- Stages 3 and 4: slow-wave sleep muscle tone is variable
- Stage 5: decrease in muscle tone; bursts of rapid eye movement; penile erections or sexual arousal in females may occur

Sleep Cycles

The hallmark of a good sleep rests on an individual being able to go through all sleep phases. Non-REM sleep often consists of two stages of light sleep which progress into the next two stages of slow-wave sleep, also known as Delta Sleep. As the closed eyelids display bursts of rapid eye movement (REM), the individual goes into a phase of deep sleep.

More stimulation and agitation is required to rouse an individual from REM sleep. Dreaming often occurs during the REM phase of sleep. A healthy individual spends about 50% of total sleep time in stage 2 sleep, about 20% in REM sleep, and the remaining 30% in the other stages. Eight hours of sleep are required by many people to permit sleep to evolve through its various stages. Much research has shown all stages of sleep to be present in healthy individuals over an average eight-hour sleep period. Only after a person has passed through all stages of sleep can he or she rightfully claim to have experienced "good quality sleep."

The Sleeping Brain Affects the Sleeping Body

In sleep, the body and the brain work in choreographed harmony, even though they sometimes appear to exhibit totally opposite actions or reactions. While the sleeping body can exist in a state of apparent "catatonic rest," the brain and other internal organs can remain on overdrive. There are several body functions that can switch on at night, e.g. nighttime secretion pf acid by the stomach due to the activation of nerves, hormones and the gastric proton pumps (acid-secreting pumps in the stomach).

During sleep, the human body is variably influenced by external stimuli. Depending on how lightly or deeply a person's sleep is, one individual can wake up to the sound of a "pin drop" but another may slumber while it thunders. It is notable that evidence exists that the brain during sleep can continue to process experiences absorbed from the environment. There are learning programs that have been designed to be used during sleep, with variable effectiveness.

Early Sleep Stages

From a condition of wakefulness, the body drifts into sleep and enters phase 1 and phase 2 of non-REM sleep. Sleep during this period can be very light. There can be some tossing and turning, and the individual can easily be roused from sleep by the slightest sound. During the initial stage of non-REM sleep, the body slows down, the brain waves adopt a rhythm that seems to lull the individual toward muscle relaxation and lowering of consciousness.

Sleep-talking can occur early in sleep, and the feeling that one is about to fall or odd occurrences like leg jerks can happen in an involuntary manner. The individuals in an early phase of sleep may find themselves either waking up from these early events that cause interruption, or they may proceed to the remaining stages of sleep.

Delta Sleep

Towards the second half of non-REM sleep (phase 3 and phase 4), the brain shows evidence of electrical activity that can be measured as delta waves. This is the "Delta phase of sleep" where delta waves in the brain alternate with short, slow waves, indicating the establishment of good sleep cycles. At this point in the sleep cycle, heart rate, blood pressure and overall body dynamics have slowed down considerably and the body can be considered "completely asleep." Individuals roused from sleep at this stage are likely to experience short-lived disorientations; and it may take a while for them to adjust to their surroundings. It is reported that abnormal events, such as bed-wetting or sleepwalking, are likely to occur in susceptible individuals during this period of Delta Sleep.

The Moving Eye Phase: Rapid Eye Movement Sleep (REM)

REM sleep brings the body to the fifth and final stage, or a condition of "deep sleep." In this stage of sleep, breathing may become rapid and somewhat irregular. Eyelids can quiver as if in a trance and the mouth often opens. Heart rate increases and blood pressure sometimes rises. At this stage in the sleep process, the brain is at its most active. Table 6 lists body experiences during REM and non-REM sleep.

Body experiences during non-REM sleep

heart rate decreases and stabilizes
breathing pace slows and becomes steady
muscles relax
blood vessels dilate
blood flow to muscles increases
blood pressure decreases
metabolic rate declines about 20% from that during wakefulness

Body experiences during REM sleep

rapid eye movements
tongue movements
muscle twitches
variation in heart rate
variation in blood pressure
variation in breathing rate
dreaming

Table 6: Changes in body functions in the two major types of sleep, non-rapid eye movement sleep (non-REM) and rapid eye movement sleep (REM)

The Sleep Phases Need to Recur Day to Day

The five-phase cycle of sleep spells good sleep and repetition of these cycles in sleep over a 24-hour period promotes health. Some sleep cycles are interrupted by sleep disorders or by events in the environment. Some sleepers never reach the later stages of sleep, especially the REM. The REM stages of sleep are modified by several prescription drugs, including "sleep drugs." Over-the-counter sleeping drugs often affect REM sleep and drug or substance abusers often have major disruptions of REM sleep. Lack of REM sleep is sleep of poor quality.

The body releases certain hormones and chemicals during sleep. One of the most important is the hormone melatonin, which is secreted at night by the pineal gland located at the back of the brain. Melatonin and other hormones balance the sleep-wake cycle. Thus, the biological clock and different phases of sleep have a biochemical basis

Sleep Functions in the Elderly

Sleep in the elderly is characterized by prolonged non-REM sleep and shorter REM or deeper forms of sleep. This shift in sleeping pattern explains why seniors complain about frequent awakenings, difficulty going back to sleep after awakening, snoring or pauses in breathing, and various types of physical discomfort. With age, the first two stages of non-REM sleep (characterized by sleep-talking) are longer, the next two phases of delta sleep (characterized by the beginning of deep sleep) become shorter. Deep slumber or (REM sleep) is similarly abbreviated. Elderly people are often easily roused from sleep, and are susceptible to minor wakening stimuli in their surroundings. The snoozing mature individual may often say, "I'm not sleeping, just closing my eyes."

Cool Kids Don't Sleep?

Many young people have self-imposed short sleep patterns and are likely to miss out on important phases of REM sleep. Some teenagers tend to think of sleep as an interruption of their social calendar. The teenage or adolescent calendar often revolves around school, friends, "hanging out" the Internet, and a weekend whirl of "malling" and "partying." A habit common among teenagers is sleeping late on school days and trying to recover missed sleep on selected days, usually the weekends. However, many youngsters and their parents do not realize the importance of the Circadian Rhythm, where going through all five phases of sleep on a regular basis, is mandatory. Good sleep habits in high school students help in learning, memory and the promotion of well-being. Experts recommend 8 to 9 hours of sleep each night for youngsters (adolescents and teens).

Perchance to Dream

Dreaming is a synthesis of visual images that are taken selectively from a series of personal events and memories. These experiences are pieced together often in an incomprehensible manner. Some of the images may be alien or unfamiliar to the dreamer. Dream sequences can be pleasant, sexual or even terrifying. There are certain characteristics of dreams that can be likened to abnormal circumstances that have occurred in the life of the dreamer. Night terrors are sometimes triggered by drug use or psychosocial disorders. One can compare the intense visual images of dreams with visual hallucinations, and real events. This latter phenomenon is like a delusional belief that is normally a hallmark of a psychosis. In dreams, one finds aberrations that have several qualities in common with symptoms of psychiatric disorders, even though the dreamer is quite sane.

Viewing dreams as analogous with symptoms of mental illness is a dark characterization of a dream, but many dreams are not as bizarre in origin as many people believe. It seems that the strangest and most dramatic dreams happen usually during deep (REM) sleep, but the majority of dreams are usually mundane and realistic experiences that have a coherent theme. Dreams can occur at any point during the five stages of sleep, but most well developed dreams occur in REM sleep.

Sleep studies have detected dreaming throughout all phases of sleep, including the transition from wakefulness to the beginning of sleep. Up to three quarters of all dreams may be recorded during phase 1 and phase 2 of non-REM sleep in some people; and up to 50% occur during phase 3 and phase 4 when the body is asleep and prepares to go into the REM sleep phase. Dreams are not always influenced by pre-sleep stimuli. For example, watching a violent movie before bedtime does not necessarily produce images of violence in dreams.

In the REM stage of sleep in healthy people, the body becomes somewhat "paralyzed" so that the individual experiencing dreams or nightmares does not tend to act on their dreams. There are individuals who have REM sleep disorder who do not experience this "body paralysis." This sleep disorder can result in behavior disorders. There are cases where the acting out of dreams has resulted in violence and personal injury. Unlike regular types of "sleepwalking", where the events most often occur in non-REM sleep, individuals with REM behavior disorders may require special medical investigations and medication to deal with their problems.

Concocting Dreams

How does the brain select the images or experiences and process them into a dream? The creation of a sequence in the brain that results in a dream is still somewhat of a mystery. However, our knowledge of how the brain functions has aided in the understanding of dreams. The brain behaves like a busy communications network during REM sleep, trafficking messages among its various structures. Many signals during sleep originate from the pons, a primitive region of the brain located toward the base of the brain. These signals travel to the brain region called the thalamus. The signals are relayed subsequently to the cerebral cortex, or the outer cortical layer of the brain that is responsible for receiving, processing and interpreting information. The cerebral cortex of the brain is responsible for higher mental functions, including coordinating movements, planning, executing emotions and other complex functions.

Thus, the cerebral cortex is critical to learning, thinking and analyzing. Dreaming appears to be the way the cerebral cortex of the brain interprets all the signals and translates them into a sequence of images that attempt to "tell a story." It remains puzzling to some scientists why the brain of a sleeping body can process such images into a coherent plot or an almost theatrical experience. The healthy brain of an awake body does not exhibit this type of "movie-making skill."

Chemical Controls of Sleep

Almost every hormone secretion or action in the body is affected by sleep and wake cycles. Hormones and other body chemicals that transmit signals to different parts of the body are the principal ways by which the environment communicates with the body and its special structures, such as the brain. Many hormones, including melatonin, prolactin, cortisol, sex hormones, prostaglandins and insulin, can be shown to rise and fall in a harmonious manner with Circadian Rhythms. Sleep disturbances are associated with disturbed hormone profiles during sleep.

Modern research has also implicated changes in the chemical transmissions in the immune system during periods of sleep. It has been noted that immunity falls with sleep deprivation. Some interesting theories have emerged about the role of bacteria in the gastrointestinal tract in the priming of immune function and the control of several body functions, in relationship to sleep. Sleep has been related to the presence of toxins produced by bacteria (endotoxin LPS).

Bacteria in the Colon Talk to the Brain?

The relationship between sleep and bacteria in the colon is one of several examples of how the digestive tract plays a major role in general health. Modern medicine has discovered the wide-reaching benefits of friendly bacteria in the colon. These friendly bacteria are referred to as probiotics (pro = for, biotics = life). Probiotics or friendly bacteria can be taken by individuals and these friendly bacteria can implant and grow in the colon, resulting in many positive health benefits. This is the practice of probiosis or probiotic theory. A more complete account of the value of probiotics for health is found in two of my earlier books (Holt S, "Natural Ways to Digestive Health," M Evans Publishers, Inc, NY, NY, 2000, and Holt S, "Digestion," Wellness Publishing, Newark, NJ, 2003).

The explanation of how bacteria in the colon are involved in sleep requires an understanding of the production of LPS (friendly toxins).

When LPS enters the body from bacteria in the colon, it triggers an immune response and part of this immune response is the secretion of chemicals that promote immune functions, such as mobilization of blood white cells. These chemicals are called "interleukins." In fact, one specific type of interleukin, known as interleukin-2, appears in response to LPS derived from bacteria. High levels of interleukin-2 are often found in states of sleeping and they are particularly prominent in people suffering from illness. Similar chemical events can occur from viral or parasitic infections. This explains, in part, why diseases can make people sleepy. Everyone has experienced the drowsiness from a good dose of influenza.

Sleep, Interleukins and Other Body Chemicals

There are many different permutations of the way in which hormones and body chemicals interact during sleep or wakefulness. In the case of illness with fever, other interleukins may increase in amount, driven by activation of the immune system (interleukin-1 and interleukin-6). Increases in these chemicals that transmit signals in the immune system and body cause a cascade of events where increases occur in other hormones, such as the sleep hormone melatonin. These cascades of body messages with chemicals and hormones can become quite complex. For example, following surges in melatonin in the early stages of sleep, the hormone prolactin appears. Prolactin is a kind of "stress hormone".

The natural hormone, melatonin, is reviewed in more detail in Chapter 6 where discussions exist about the formulation of the natural, dietary supplement product Sleep Naturally™ (www.naturesbenefit.com).

Surges in melatonin secretion, from a tiny gland at the back of the brain called the pineal gland, occur in 24-hour cycles in healthy people. This surge is followed by prolactin hormone secretion from the pituitary gland, located in the front lower portion of the brain. The pituitary gland secretes a number of hormones and acts like a conductor of the orchestra of endocrine glands of the body.

Sex hormone secretions change during sleep in both men and

women, particularly estrogen, progesterone and testosterone. These changes in sex hormones occur "in sync" with the secretion of insulin and growth hormones. All of these hormonal "ups and downs" are controlled by timing mechanisms in certain areas of the brain.

One important area of the brain that acts as a "timer switch" is the hypothalamus, an area of the brain found immediately above the pituitary gland. In simple terms, the hypothalamus takes information from the environment through the brain and passes it on to the "band leader" (the pituitary gland) of the endocrine orchestra (adrenal glands, thyroid glands, sex glands, etc.). The individual players in the orchestra are all endocrine glands which have their own hormones that have many different functions in the body. This complex series of events is the basis of the "harmony of life."

What is the Significance of Hormone and Chemical Changes With Sleep?

Clearly, the chemistry of life is controlled to a major degree by hormones and messenger chemicals that tell body cells to do certain things. There are many simple examples of how certain hormones work. For example, insulin tells many cells in the body to take up glucose, but it also gives powerful messages to the body to store fat, make cholesterol and raise blood pressure. One can now see a chain of events that explains why sleep disturbances cause disease.

Take the example of insulin. Sleep deprivation causes resistance to the actions of the hormone insulin, even in healthy people. Given insulin's role in weight control, blood pressure and blood cholesterol regulation, one can see how changes in the "wrong direction," when it comes to insulin, may favor the development of common diseases, such as cardiovascular disease. It has been proposed that high levels of insulin, in the presence of resistance to the actions of the hormone insulin on blood glucose, may lead to heart disease, diabetes and cancer (Holt S, "Combat Syndrome X, Y and Z....," Wellness Publishing, Newark, NJ, 2002).

The modern epidemic of Syndrome X is linked to sleeplessness which is linked to other factors such as stress. Recent studies in more than 4,000 schoolchildren have linked stress with obesity. While stress may tend cause children to eat more, it also causes sleep deprivation. The researchers in these recent studies of stress and obesity in children have tended to focus their conclusions on calorie intake. I believe that sleep deprivation plays a role in obesity. The whole situation is a vicious cycle because stress aggravates the components of Syndrome X and contributes to their ability to damage health.

The concepts that I am attempting to explain may seem unduly complex to people without medical or health care training, but I want people to persist to understand the widespread ramifications of sleep deprivation. Let us take another example of how hormone imbalance due to sleep problems could cause diseases. If there is any single hormone secretion that dominates the hormone profile of the female body it is estrogen. Body functions become "screwed-up" with estrogen imbalances, e.g. menopause and PMS. For example, if high levels of certain sex hormones, such as estrogen, occur without the balance of other sex hormones, such as progesterone, then symptoms of estrogen excess can occur. This situation results in bloating, feeling of abdominal fullness and even weight gain. Notice how these symptoms are similar to premenstrual syndrome or the modern diagnostic category of pre-menstrual disorders (PMD). I have found in my clinical experience that many young females with premenstrual syndrome (PMS) are sleep deprived. Few individuals with PMS can consider the fact that their symptoms could be, in part, related to their poor sleeping habits.

Even more sinister results can occur from the dominance of one sex hormone. Estrogen causes body tissues to grow and if present without balance, then it can contribute to the development of cancer; especially cancers that are dependent upon estrogen, such as breast cancer. Thus, the end results of losing hormone balance from losing sleep are much more of a concern than many people, including health care givers, may have realized.

New Discoveries: Hypocretin, The Anti-Sleep Hormone?

By studying dogs with narcolepsy that fall asleep "at will", scientists have identified a hormone deficiency that causes sleep. This hormone is called hypocretin or orexin. Narcolepsy is a condition characterized by excessive, repeated lapses into sleep. This condition affects about 1 in 2,000 people in the population and it may be caused by a lack of the hormone hypocretin (orexin).

Research leading to the discovery of this master "anti-sleep hormone" was undertaken by Dr. Emmanuel Mignot, M.D. and his colleagues in a group of Doberman pinscher dogs with narcolepsy. These dogs had a deficiency of the hormone hypocretin. While the role of hypocretin in sleep and other body functions is not completely understood, it appears that this hormone affects the key neurotransmitters (brain chemicals, serotonin and dopamine) that control sleep and wakefulness.

Serotonin and dopamine cause brain activation and they are modulated by natural agents (see Sleep Naturally™, www.sleepnaturally.com). The activity of other hormones, such as melatonin, growth hormone, insulin, cortisol and glucogen, etc., are altered during sleep cycles and the story of sleep is not just down to one hormone. However, further characterization of the actions of hypocretin (orexin) may lead to better ways of inducing restful sleep in the insomniac, or relief from excessive sleep in the narcoleptic.

Chapter Summary

Major advances have been made in the scientific study of sleep and wakefulness. Much of this science has focused on the relationship between the brain and the body during sleep. There are many other changes in body functions during sleep that are beginning to unravel. Beyond changes in the nervous system are adaptations in body chemistry and, in particular, alterations in hormone secretions and the actual function of hormones. While changes in sleep patterns can be linked to changes in measurements of several body functions, there are a number of disturbances during sleep that defy simple explanation.

The science of sleep is evolving and new specialties are developing as various activities during sleep become the focus of attention. One fertile area of research is the interpretation of dreams, but this area of sleep research is not subject to a consensus of opinion. What dreams mean and how they affect well-being remains unclear. The science of sleep is finding widespread application in specialized sleep centers. These centers of medical excellence are discovering the harmony of body function and its relationships with sleep cycles.

Chapter 4:

HEALTH CONSEQUENCES OF LACK OF SLEEP

An Introduction to Sleep Deprivation

What happens to the body that does not get enough sleep has been likened to an overstressed automobile engine. The overworked engine loses "steam," sputters, and then wears out. Old cars tend to wear out quicker, but a new (younger) car could probably be resurrected by a simple "tune up." In an analogous manner, elderly people who are deprived of sleep find it hard to recover, but a teenager with a sleep debt can recover faster than an adult. Disabilities and even death can result from serious insomnia, especially in the elderly. The old person who wakes at night and wanders in the house may be prone to accidents and falls which often cause fractures. The fracture of a hip in the elderly is a major negative milestone in the elderly (www.antiporosis.com). Moreover, a young brain that is deprived of sleep may not undergo a full maturation process necessary for its proper functioning. In addition, the uncommon circumstance of sleep deprivation in infants is a sinister cause of "failure to thrive."

More than one half of elderly people with insomnia admit to having difficulty handling stress, concentrating and making decisions. These problems can occur in the elderly at home or in nursing facilities. In population surveys, the elderly often seek relief from sleeplessness through reading, watching TV, exercise and simple acts like drinking a glass of milk. Others resort to extremes by either taking sleeping medications or suffering in silence. It is clear that many elderly people with insomnia do not receive appropriate interventions for their sleeplessness.

A recent study at the University of Pittsburgh School of Medicine suggested that older people (from 59 to 91 years) who had "normal sleep" lived longer, while those who suffered continuous disruptions to their sleep are accident-prone and more likely to die earlier. The study recommended lifestyle changes and behavioral therapy for senior citizens who cannot sleep. The advice included several lifestyle changes, such as creating a safe environment for a restful sleep, avoidance of excessive caffeine and alcohol intake before bedtime and limiting afternoon naps.

The Young Sleepers

In children and teenagers, significant lack of sleep invariably results in some form of emotional disturbance and poor physical or mental performance. This poor performance can result in anxiety and can contribute to a number of psychological problems or psychiatric illnesses in young people. Several studies have shown that "sleepy students" often exhibit mediocre performance in school and this may result in academic failure. The reduction in the efficiency of daily tasks of some teenagers may be quite subtle. The sleep-deprived child or teenager cannot memorize efficiently and has difficulty in focusing on many issues that determine their ability to learn. Considerable problems exist for sleep-deprived youngsters when they are doing more than one thing at once (multi-tasking). Abstract thought is extinguished in the poor sleeper.

The sleep-deprived young person is often easily distracted and frustrated. They may become demoralized to the extent that they engage in antisocial behavior. In order to mask their frustrations, students with insomnia may behave in an unpredictable and apparently contrarian manner by exhibiting intermittent periods of excitement and poor concentration, otherwise referred to as "hyperactivity." I believe that sleep deprivation in children and young teenagers is an overlooked cause of what has become the common diagnosis of attention deficit disorder (ADD). Furthermore, I believe that attention deficit disorder is overdiagnosed and overtreated with drugs that have mood-changing effects and a tendency to develop dependence (addiction). Drugs used to treat ADD often upset sleep patterns.

In summary, sleep deprivation can result in extreme behavioral aberrations ranging from impulsive behavior to frank depression. Parents and teachers may label a child as "spinning out of control" without the simple realization that poor sleep is the root of the problem.

Sleep and Learning

I have stressed repeatedly that the later stages of a normal sleep cycle are obligatory for good mental function during the day, especially in relationship to learning skills and the retention of memory. Eight hours of sleep have been shown to be, on average, helpful in facilitating, especially in youngsters and young adults, the learning process. A research study by Dr. Robert Stickgold M.D. and his colleagues at the Harvard Medical School showed that approximately eight hours of sleep are required to develop new physical and mental skills, such as learning a new sport or learning to play a musical instrument. The studies of Stickgold and his colleagues confirm other findings that a well-rested brain can process new information and memorize events with efficiency.

It has been noted that during the first 2 hours of slow-wave type sleep, much new information are stored in the memory regions of the brain and processed in the higher centers of the brain. During the intermediate stages of sleep (about a four-hour period), the brain engages in a kind of internal dialogue within itself. In simplistic terms, the brain sorts out newly acquired information and distributes this information into other regions of the brain, where it becomes imprinted. In later phases of sleep (the last two hours or so of sleep), the higher centers of the brain (cerebral cortex) engage in active dreaming. Furthermore, the brain reviews or reenacts much of the newly acquired information and skills rather like a rehearsal for a play. Ultimately, the information is stored in the memory banks of the brain for later recall.

Sleep in Children

Tots and toddlers are often encouraged to take regular periods of sleep in daycare centers and some primary schools. This is a healthy practice that should be encouraged. The importance of regular sleep should be emphasized during the teaching of young children. Sleep should be portrayed to youngsters as a pleasurable event. Unfortunately, some parents may threaten a child with an early bedtime. This parental act should be extinguished and for a young child, the idea of going to bed must not be linked with any form of punitive activity.

Every parent is familiar with "bedtime hassles" from their kids. The "bedtime hassle" often starts during the "terrible twos." While there are uncommon occurrences of serious sleep disorders in children, most sleep problems in the age groups 2 years to 14 years are related to poor routines and lack of positive discipline. Any sign of a sleep disorder in an infant or baby must be taken very seriously and medication of children with anything, including dietary supplements, must be avoided without expert supervision by a medical practitioner. That said, I believe that sleeping pills, be them drugs or supplements, have little, if any, role in individuals below the age of 18 years.

The common, garden-variety of sleep disorder in children (age range of 2 and 14 years) can be corrected by structuring daily routines in "a clever manner." The key to success is to understand the motivation and desires of the child, who will not go to bed, go to sleep or stay asleep. In other words, parents must learn to outsmart their kids and negotiate in a gentle manner. The young child has powers of observation and interpretation of events that are far more sophisticated than parents believe. The toddler sees the pressure to go to bed as an event in their life where adults are removing their presence. In some cases, separation anxiety operates. The will of a healthy child between the ages of 2 and 4 years must be respected, as must the determination of the "know-all teenager." Again, I stress the notion of applying discipline in a positive manner, with rewards for structured activity.

Many self-help books discuss problems in the sleeping habits of kids, but few give practical suggestions. I shall give an example of structuring that can be successful in breaking the "stop-up habits" of some kids. After the age of 3 years, kids can understand daily routines. Certain ordered rituals prior to going to bed are important for children. Selecting clothes to wear the next day, placing toys in order in their rooms, etc. are activities that bypass the perception by the child that they are being abandoned at bedtime.

"Sleepyheads from stop-up routines" must not be rewarded. Children capable of assisting in dressing themselves in the morning will be very responsive to the events preceding bedtime. If routines are broken, they cannot be rewarded. Simple structuring of day-to-day activity is a powerful way of breaking "sleep hassles". There are obvious things for parents to avoid. A baby or child brought to a marital bed will remain with more determination than any albatross following a ship. If a parent makes a bed with a young child, then they should expect to be in for a big fight when the child needs to sleep in their own room. Kids in marital beds can place great stresses on spousal relationships.

I reiterate my earlier warnings that drug or natural sleeping products are not for use in children and they should be avoided in pregnancy, when breastfeeding or in the active phases of attempting to conceive. Behavioral therapy for sleep disorders has to be preferred in childhood and pregnancy.

Reviewing the Litany of Sleep Disorders

A large proportion of Western society suffers from one form or another of sleep disorder. On a regular basis, sleep scientists come out with new descriptions of specific sleep disorders. It is useful to review some of the many types of sleep disorders that have been described. Table 7 summarizes a variety of sleep disorders.

Type of Sleep Disorder	Some Causes/ Comments
Insomnia	Psychiatric and medical disease, medications, poor nutrition, environmental factors, poor lifestyle, simple anxiety, substance abuse and ignorance about sleep hygiene
Daytime sleepiness	Affects one in 20 in the population, has many different causes, major physical and mental disability can be experienced
Sleep apneas	They come in two basic types, central sleep apnea and obstructive sleep apnea. Central types are caused by brain disease or disorder in the young or elderly and heart failure. Obstructive sleep apnea is caused by anything that narrows the upper airway or impaired thyroid function (hypothyroidism).

Leg discomforts and movements	The common condition of restless leg syndrome is associated with periodic movements of the legs or arms in sleep. This disorder tends to run in families and as many as one in three elderly people have this disorder. The restless leg syndrome can result in symptoms or signs in a person during wakefulness or sleep, and it is sometimes referred to as the "crazy leg" disorder. Afflicted people may have all kinds of different sensations in their legs with jerky movements of their legs over which they can exert little control. There are special diagnostic procedures to detect these disorders.
Abnormal behavior from sleep	These disorders are sometimes called parasomnias. Even restful sleep can be associated with abnormal behavior that may or not may not wake the individual. Arousal disorders include sleepwalking, confusional episodes and sleep terrors, somewhat more common in children. Nightmares often result in awakenings but they are not usually associated with episodes of confusion or abnormal sleep behavior. Abnormal behaviors that result from sleep occur during various sleep cycles and other activities may occur, such as bed wetting (nocturnal enuresis) and episodes of sexual arousal, including penile erection and even orgasm.

Table 7: A discussion of different sleep disorders and their causes.

Sleep Apnea

Perhaps the most significant sleep disorder that may be associated with diseases and even risks of premature death is the sleep problem called sleep apnea. Sleep apnea is among the commonest reasons for a person to receive a detailed evaluation in a sleep center. The word apnea has its origins in the Greek language. "Apnea" means literally "without breath" or "without wind." In other words, people who periodically stop breathing during sleep to a variable degree, fall into this category of sleep apnea. Perhaps the commonest association of sleep apnea is excessive snoring.

So important is the condition of sleep apnea that it has been specifically classified by sleep scientists into different types of sleep abnormalities. Sleep apneas are a variety of breathing problems during sleep and they are, by far, the most serious problems that affect sleep patterns. There are fundamentally two types of sleep apnea. One is called "central apnea," where there is a cessation of breathing from within the body or brain and the other principal type is "obstructive apnea." As the name suggests, obstructive apnea is due to a blocking of the upper airways in the presence of continuous breathing activity.

The acts of not breathing or obstructed breathing result in lack of oxygenation to the body tissues and fragmentation of sleep. These circumstances have wide-ranging effects on health and may even contribute to heart failure, as well as their readily detectable effects on brain functions, such as thought and memory. About one in 20 women and as many as one in 10 men may have a degree of significant sleep apnea. These population statistics are startling!

Notes on the Medical Management of Sleep Apnea

Effective treatment of sleep apnea is important to reduce disability and prevent death. There must be a correct matching of the severity of sleep apnea with the intensity of treatment. Individuals with few symptoms and no co-existing disease can be followed with simple advice on lifestyle change. Advice on weight control is one of the most important interventions in the treatment of sleep apnea. Patients who have severe diseases, such as degenerative disorders of the nervous system or advanced lung disease, have the worst prognosis and they require special management.

The treatment of sleep apnea has been revolutionized by the use of assisted breathing at night using a device that delivers continuous positive pressure to the airways (CPAP). This positive airway pressure using CPAP is a mainstay in the management of obstructive sleep apnea. There are surgical approaches to deal with obstructed airways, but these interventions are decreasing in popularity.

Dentists are making significant contributions to the management of sleep apnea and some dental appliances are quite effective in keeping the upper airways open in the person with obstructive sleep apnea. Some drugs have been tried for the treatment of sleep apnea, but they have not been beneficial overall. Significant degrees of sleep apnea should not be self-managed and the avoidance of all substances that may suppress breathing is advisable in established cases of sleep apnea.

Sleep Apnea and Obesity

There is no doubt that sleep apnea is more common in people who are overweight or obese. There are typical characteristics of individuals who have obstructive sleep apnea. These people are usually middle aged or elderly men with moderate obesity and many have Syndrome X (obesity combined with high blood pressure, high cholesterol and intolerance to glucose in the diet or insulin resistance). Central types of sleep apnea tend to occur in the very young and the elderly. Most cases of severe sleep apnea are found in infants or the elderly (average age of 70 years). On occasion, central apnea, where breathing does not occur, results from severe diseases of the central nervous system, such as cerebrovascular disease and other degenerative neurological conditions.

Spotting Sleep Apnea

Sleep apnea is quite easy for the casual observer to spot. However, the detection of sleep apnea requires direct observation of the individual during sleep. There is a set of criteria that some doctors use to make a definite diagnosis of sleep apnea. In general terms, any person who stops breathing more than 10 times in one hour, for at least a period of 10 seconds, can be assumed to have sleep apnea. This type of sleep apnea requires careful and expert management by a medical practitioner. The definitive diagnosis of sleep apnea requires a well-planned sleep study which can only be performed in an "accredited sleep center."

Evolving Insomnia and Drugs

Insomnia is the most common form of sleep disturbance. Most people associate insomnia with shortened duration of sleep, but sleep quality is just as important as sleeping times. There are a host of factors that initiate or aggravate poor sleep. Several can be explained by medical or psychiatric illness, but most often sleep disturbance is linked to simple emotional upset. However, several drugs and diseases can cause episodes of insomnia.

Both stimulant and sedating drugs can affect sleeping patterns in many ways. Major imbalances in sleep have been recorded with the use of anti-hypertensive drugs, bronchodilators, corticosteroids, anti-arrhythmic medications, calcium channel blockers, anti-Parkinsonian drugs, anticonvulsant medicine, anti-depressants, non-steroidal anti-inflammatory drugs and even hypnotic drugs used to promote sleep. The idea that "it may be your drugs" when it comes to insomnia, should be a prominent thought.

There are many other medications that interfere with sleep and many are freely available for purchase over the counter (OTC), including allergy medications, slimming tablets and even dietary supplements that have weight loss claims. A common cause of sleeplessness in the 1990s was the widespread use of ephedra (ma huang) in dietary supplements used for weight control.

Dangerous Weight Control Tactics and Sleep Disturbance

Ephedra is not a safe substance when used inappropriately and it has been abused in individuals who believed that it could boost aerobic fitness. There is a modern trend to heavily promote "non-ephedra" alternatives in dietary supplements for weight control. However, non-ephedra, natural products such as synephrine (Citrus aurantium) can interfere with sleep and whether or not they are safer than ephedra remains to be seen. These non-ephedra slimming ingredients can raise blood pressure, but they do not have the same central nervous stimulating effects of ephedra. In brief, this means that these "ephedra alternatives" are probably not as effective in weight control as ephedra.

Weight control has to be primarily planned for general health. Weight loss tactics that ignore general health should be avoided. There is no "quick fix" for weight, despite the promises of marketing predators. The key to weight control is the consumption of a healthy, calorie-controlled diet, behavior modification and exercise. Certainly, the restriction of simple sugars in the diet has produced promising results in weight control programs. These low carbohydrate diets or lifestyles are quite popular and they may be a good basis for the combat against Syndrome X (www.combatsyndromex.com). Syndrome X is the combination of being overweight with high blood pressure and high blood cholesterol, all linked by underlying resistance to the hormone insulin. Insulin resistance leads to glucose intolerance.

Among the causes of Syndrome X are abnormal sleep patterns; and components of Syndrome X, especially obesity, can contribute to significant sleep disorders, such as sleep apnea. I have discussed these matters in more detail earlier in this book (See Chapter 1 and Chapter 2). For a detailed review of the major public health importance of the metabolic Syndrome X, I refer readers to my two books on the subject (Holt S, "Combat Syndrome X, Y and Z...", Wellness Publishing, Newark, NJ, 2002 and Holt S and Wright J, "Syndrome X Nutritional Factors," Wellness Publishing, Newark, NJ, 2003, www.combatsyndromex.com).

In my writings, I have cautioned people about the use of dietary supplements that have "alleged" effects on increasing body metabolism and "fat burning". There are 70 million Americans who have Syndrome X characterized by the variable combination of obesity, hypertension, hypercholesterolemia and insulin resistance. Key factors in the cause of Syndrome X are the messages given by excess circulating insulin to store fat, make cholesterol and raise blood pressure. It seems nonsensical to have people use drugs or supplements that raise blood pressure in the face of increased risks of hypertension or the established presence of hypertension. Syndrome X is, in my opinion, a contraindication to the use of ephedra, ephedra-free supplements and any "slimming drug." Please bear in mind that this means that as many as 70 million Americans have a contraindication or relative contraindication to these "stimulating drugs" or dietary supplements.

Ephedra Deaths

I believe that several of the deaths reported with the use of ephedra have resulted from the inappropriate use of this dietary supplement in people with Syndrome X. A particularly dangerous use of ephedra is for a person with elevated blood pressure or Syndrome X to combine ephedra use with rigorous exercise. This combination has resulted in stroke and death from heart attack. It has also resulted in the recent solicitation of lawsuits on TV by America's many lawyers.

These are compelling reasons for regulation of the use of ephedra. However, it would be a shame for ephedra to lose its status as a dietary supplement because it has very valuable benefits in sinus and respiratory disorders in selected people. It surprises me that ephedra-containing dietary supplements and "ephedra substitute" dietary supplements are still the most popular of all dietary supplements. The promise of a "quick-fix" for weight control is an unfulfilled promise and I reiterate that global health must be the fundamental basis of controlling America's obesity problem.

Low Carbohydrate Diets and Lifestyle

I support the restriction of simple sugars as a mainstay in dietary approaches to weight control. However, diets such as the Atkins, Carbohydrate Addicts and Zone Diets are not enough when used alone. The Atkins Diet works for about a six- to twelve-month period only. What makes the difference is to use nutritional ways of "blunting" surges in blood glucose and secondarily "blunting" rises in blood insulin. This approach facilitates the effectiveness of low carbohydrate diets or lifestyles. This approach makes the difference when added to the dietary restriction of simple sugars and it helps prevent the common and very unfortunate weight gain that can follow the use of a low carbohydrate diet (www.combatsyndromex.com, www.lowcarbx.com, www.lowcarbohydratedietfacilitator.com).

I have developed a group of nutritional products which provide nutritional support for several aspects of the natural combat against Syndrome X (Syndrome X Nutritional Factors™, www.naturesbenefit.com). In addition, the use of nutritional agents that complement low carbohydrate diets, such as Low Carbohydrate Diet Facilitator™, may be helpful and make a difference to the health benefit and effectiveness of a low carbohydrate lifestyle.

Simple Sugars and Sleep

How is the handling of simple sugar by the body relevant to sleep patterns? In general terms, excessive consumption of simple sugars in the diet causes rapid swings in blood insulin. This circumstance may result in an overswing of blood glucose to the downside. This is a condition called hypoglycemia (low blood sugar). Episodes of low blood sugar have been associated with insomnia and periodic awakening during the night. In addition, hypoglycemia is known to be associated with daytime and nocturnal food cravings.

Recently, scientists have attempted to describe a series of sleep disorders that they have called "nocturnal eating disorders". One may see how a poor diet with excessive refined sugar can be linked to a whole host of interconnecting medical problems including sleep disorders and Syndrome X.

A real worry is that Syndrome X is a common forerunner to maturity onset diabetes mellitus and Syndrome X constitutes a primary group of risk factors for cardiovascular diseases – the U.S. nation's number one cause of death. Furthermore, Syndrome X has been associated with a wide variety of diseases including, but not limited to: irregular menstruation, polycystic ovary syndrome (PCOS), fatty liver, sleep disturbance, chronic inflammatory disease, infertility and cancer (Holt S, "Combat Syndrome X, Y and Z...," Wellness Publishing, Newark, NJ, 2002).

Excessive Daytime Sleepiness, Obesity and Syndrome X

Excessive daytime sleepiness is a common problem in all age groups. A particularly severe form of daytime sleepiness is called narcolepsy where people fall asleep at will. Other forms of daytime sleepiness can be graded in a severity. When it occurs with repetitive tasks, it is mild, but when someone falls asleep during an interview, significant problems must be presumed to be present. There has been a major increase in daytime sleepiness that is associated with obesity. This is due to the increasing occurrence of weight gain in the U.S. population.

Obesity and somnolence go "hand in hand" and they have been labeled as part of a disorder called "the Pickwickian Syndrome," after the famous Charles Dickens character. While being overweight and sleepy may often go together, it is not generally realized that this is a dangerous combination and it can herald the onset of high blood pressure and cardiac disease in some people. People with excessive daytime sleepiness due to sleep deprivation may not be aware that they have a sleeping disorder, until they exhibit disturbing signs. Such symptoms and signs include: forgetfulness, inattentiveness, irritability or fatigue. Again, one can see the inextricable linkage between sleep disorders and aspects of the Metabolic Syndrome X where cardiovascular risks and death or disability from many causes can result (www.sleepnaturally.com, www.combatsyndromex.com).

Parasomnias

Parasomnias form a group of significant health problems. These parasomnias (para = beside, somnia = sleep) are quite common in medical practice. Arousal disorders or parasomnias can induce reactions severe enough to force individuals out of their beds, and they can result in physical activity during varying depths of sleep. Children are particularly vulnerable to these types of sleep disturbances which are exhibited often in the form of sleepwalking, sleep terrors or arousals from sleep in a state of confusion. Adults also experience parasomnias. One common example is repeated episodes of leg movements called the "restless leg syndrome." This condition is quite common in the elderly and it can be very difficult to treat.

It is estimated that about 18% of the U.S. population have problems with sleepwalking or other nocturnal behavior which are most often benign events. However, when sleepwalking occurs in association with behavioral aberrations or sleep terrors, it may cause the individual to act on irrational impulses. An effective way to deal with sleepwalking is not to arouse sleeping individuals, but to guide them quietly back to their beds, so that they can resume normal sleep. Sleepwalking must be managed by a sleep expert.

People who find themselves disoriented when they wake up may be experiencing a condition called " confusional arousal." These individuals are often not fully awake, but they are capable of physical activity. Reflex movements in a state of confusion can be quite dangerous. When they occur in the elderly, they can cause accidents. Nightmares may occur when the sleeper is in the later stage of sleep (REM sleep), particularly if he or she is engaged in dreaming, but most nightmares are not "acted out" by the disturbed sleeper..

Disruptions to the Circadian Rhythm

I have emphasized repeatedly that the body functions with its own inbuilt clock. From early childhood, humankind develops certain rhythms that play a major role in many body functions. This form of "body programming" signals people when to sleep at night and when to wake up in the morning. These cycles of activity usually coincide with night-and-day or light-and-dark periods. These well developed biological cycles are also known as Circadian Rhythms which are heavily influenced by many factors, including personal habits, cultural factors and the external environment. Certainly, these biological rhythms are orchestrated by the brain and have rhythmicity over a period of about 24 to 25 hours.

Disruptions to the Circadian Rhythm have significant social, behavioral, medical and psychological outcomes. Individuals who experience changes in their "inbuilt body clock" are sometimes prone to disorientation. These people manifest their problems during the day time by committing errors, becoming momentarily indecisive or developing memory lapses. Their behavioral problems are typified by experiencing difficulty in focusing on multiple tasks that they should be quite capable of performing. For example, individuals with a disruption of their biological rhythm can experience difficulty in driving a vehicle or operating machinery. They may become a public danger because they are not able to react efficiently to unexpected events. These victims of disordered body rhythm have poor ability to concentrate and like most sleep-deprived people, they become prone to emotional and psychological stress. This can develop into a "vicious cycle."

The most common disorders associated with a disruption of the Circadian Rhythm include:

"Delayed Sleep Phase Syndrome". This disorder is characterized by difficulty in falling asleep at night and difficulty in waking up in the morning. It is a particular problem in young people who go to bed late at night, but are forced to wake up at an early hour with regularity. Many people may attempt to reset their Circadian Rhythms by catching up on sleep during weekends, but they may find themselves poorly prepared for the toils of a regular Monday.

"Advanced Sleep Phase Syndrome". This disorder is essentially the opposite of Delayed Sleep Phase Syndrome. An individual experiences overwhelming sleepiness early in the evening, usually around 6 p.m. It is associated with waking up much too early in the morning, between 1 a.m. and 3 a.m. Thus, individuals who sleep earlier than their regular bedtime schedules can end up with early morning wakening at times much earlier than they wish to surface. These people can lie awake, struggling with the inability to go back to sleep.

"Jet Lag" is familiar to almost everyone and it is usually caused when one travels to a destination with a different time zone. The body and mind are placed in a circumstance which forces adjustments to time differences. In Chapter 6, the role of body hormones in sleep regulation and adjustments is discussed in some detail (See Melatonin). Body adjustments to jet lag occur over much slower periods than most individuals realize. For example, traveling through time zones amounting to 12 hours can exert their main disabling effects three days after arriving at a destination and in some people it can take more than two weeks to fully adjust Circadian Rhythms to a 12-hour difference in time zones.

"Shift Sleepers" — shifts in work schedules cause another form of disruption of biological rhythms, akin to jet lag. Problems occur when day and night shifts are rapidly reversed and particular problems can occur when frequent changes in working time occur over extended periods of time. Shift workers can have some of the most confused or bizarre biological rhythms.

Chapter Summary

This chapter has illustrated the far-reaching negative consequences of sleep disturbances on general health. Sleeplessness and its sequelae cross all age and social boundaries. Poor sleep is a contributory cause to many different illnesses ranging from simple behavioral problems to potential contribution to chronic diseases, such as heart disease, cancer and diabetes mellitus. There are many sleep disorders. Some disorders, such as sleep apnea, must be taken very seriously and managed in an expert manner. There are many reasons to look for natural ways to promote healthy sleep and such pathways must be further examined (www.sleepnaturally.com).

Chapter 5:

A LITANY OF SLEEP AIDS

The Use of Sleeping Pills

Modern physicians are attempting to educate themselves on the science of sleep, but many doctors remain unfamiliar with basic sleep and dream cycles; and they may be even less familiar with the effect of sleeping pills on the quality and even the duration of sleep. Studies in clinical practice reveal that many doctors do not even ask patients how they slept, even after they took a prescribed sleeping pill or after the physician had withdrawn the "sleeping pill" from a patient. It is well known that the use or withdrawal of a wide variety of drugs can produce sleep alterations and distressing symptoms.

Many sleeping drugs suppress REM sleep and they will suppress dreaming. There is often an increase in REM sleep following the withdrawal of sleeping pills. Associated with this phenomenon is a frequent increase in the intensity of dreaming and the development of alarming episodes of insomnia. Rebound insomnia is a huge problem when many popular sleeping drugs are withdrawn. This type of rebound insomnia has not been observed to any major degree when natural agents such as herbs and nutrients are used to facilitate sleep (www.sleepnaturally.com). Rebound insomnia is a common under-reported consequence of over-the-counter sleeping drugs, such as antihistamines. Pharmaceutical companies argue that newer, short acting sleeping pills are less likely to cause side effects, but the jury remains out.

Some Aspects of Hypnotic Drugs

Much medical literature states that drugs for sleep are best used in selected individuals. However, many over-the-counter drugs for sleep are available and prescriptions for hypnotic drugs are often "repeated" without "repeated" evaluation of the patient. There is no doubt that the use of pharmaceuticals for sleep is best combined with an integrated medical approach that includes lifestyle and behavioral change.

There may be some benefits to the use of hypnotic medications during temporary periods of stress or other disturbances of routines such as travel or major changes in work schedules. While drugs work to put people to sleep, so do many natural agents that are reviewed in detail in Chapter 6 (Sleep Naturally, www.sleepnaturally.com). Many physicians aim to prescribe the lowest effective dose of a sleeping tablet, but this approach is not necessarily safe because dependence on "hypnotic" drugs may develop quite quickly.

Disadvantages of Drugs for Sleep

There are a wide variety of drugs that will help an individual to sleep, but many of these drugs carry disadvantages and limitations. The most commonly used drugs for sleep include: over-the-counter antihistamine products, prescription benzodiazepines and sometimes antidepressant drugs. There are other very effective drugs to induce sleep but they have generally been abandoned in routine clinical practice. These obsolete sleeping drugs include barbiturates and related compounds which are quite dangerous when taken in excess.

Effective marketing of over-the-counter (OTC) sleeping aids, such as antihistamines, has resulted in their widespread use. However, these drugs are quite limited in their ability to induce sleep compared with other drugs. Furthermore, these OTC drugs may be less effective than natural, nutritional agents that can induce sleep, such as herbs, botanicals and selected nutrients. Antihistamine drugs are long-acting and often produce hangover effects. These drugs interfere with certain types of nerves in the body called cholinergic nerves and this often results in temporary blurred vision, a dry mouth and dry mucus membranes.

The "kings" of pharmaceuticals include a group of drugs called benzodiazepines that are often used as hypnotic medications. Benzodiazepines have different duration of effect, but they are all rapidly absorbed and relatively quick in their onset. These drugs are sometimes not handled very well by elderly people and confusional episodes from the use of sleeping tablets are a common problem in the elderly. The benzodiazepines that act for short periods of time are to be preferred over those that act for longer periods of time, because the longer acting types of benzodiazepines can cause excessive daytime sleepiness. The use of these drugs has been linked to accidents and injuries especially in the elderly.

Benzodiazepine drugs can be used under close supervision with some benefit in people who have significant anxiety disorders. While the shorter acting types of hypnotic drugs may cause less drowsiness during the day, they are a particularly common cause of rebound wakefulness and withdrawal symptoms when they are discontinued. The popular drug zolpidem (Ambien®) is not a benzodiazepine and it is short acting. However, it is not devoid of an ability to cause rebound withdrawal symptoms. Perhaps, the most severe rebound insomnia is experienced when there is a sudden cessation of taking the drug triazolam, a benzodiazepine. One particularly unpleasant side effect of triazolam is the occurrence of anterograde amnesia. This means loss of memory prior to taking the medication. Memory loss can be quite alarming in mature individuals. Table 8 lists some side effects of hypnotic drugs, especially benzodiazepines.

Dizziness	Rebound anxiety
Headache	Rebound inability to sleep
Behavior change	Amnesia
Loss of balance	Interaction with other drugs
Slurred speech	Development of dependence
Confusion	Mixed drug abuse
Hangover	Interaction with some sleep disorders

Table 8: A list of side effects that may be noted in people taking drugs to help them sleep. Many of these side effects are described with the use of benzodiazepines. Drugs, such as barbiturates, can be quite dangerous and may, for example, interfere with breathing during sleep. All medications to induce sleep are to be used with the utmost care in people with liver, kidney or lung disease; and they should not be taken during pregnancy or during breastfeeding. Other serious but less common side effects have been

described with sleeping tablets which are often used in suicide attempts. Anti-depressant drugs that are sedating are best reserved for the patient with depression and these drugs have an extensive list of potential side effects.

Dangers From the Prolonged Use of Sleeping Drugs

Individuals with chronic insomnia are advised to seek expert medical care. I am not attempting to give advice to people with major sleep disturbances or encourage people to self-medicate. People with major sleep disorders are encouraged to talk to their physicians about "coming off," or at least, reducing the dose of sleeping medications. It has been my experience, in uncontrolled but direct observations, that some people who are hooked on sleeping pills can benefit from natural ways to facilitate sleep, using guidelines of behavior modification and natural, dietary supplements that are proposed in the Sleep Naturally Plan.

Several studies have shown that the withdrawal of pharmaceuticals used to induce sleep can result in severe adverse clinical disturbances. It is somewhat scary to note that such disturbances have been described in some people after they have taken certain sleeping tablets for only a couple of weeks. This is especially the case if such people took hypnotic drugs on a regular basis. Characteristic adverse reactions to the withdrawal of several sleeping drugs include: nightmares, inability to fall asleep, inability to stay asleep, anxiety, depression and a residual feeling that they have slept poorly, even though they may have slept with reasonable duration, but questionable quality.

Clearly, if people are seeking adjuncts (extra aids) to sleep then they should exercise the simplest and gentlest approaches first. These approaches form the basis of the Sleep Naturally Plan and involve many potential easy lifestyle changes and the appropriate use of natural dietary supplements (www.sleepnaturally.com).

Revising Expectations: A Key to a Good Slumber

Insomnia can cause a learned behavior, where going to bed can be dreaded or at least be anxiety-provoking. Wrestling with the idea of a poor night's sleep can become a self-fulfilling prophecy for many people. To attempt to sleep in the presence of this kind of self-induced anxiety is rewarded with wakefulness that is plagued with torment.

Duke University researchers studied the value of educating people with sleep problems about their negative attitudes to going to sleep. These scientists found that modifying behavior and attitudes to sleep result in a beneficial outcome. With education and insight, individuals with insomnia can sleep better and longer. Other studies have confirmed similar benefits of behavior modification and change of thought patterns regarding sleep. These approaches are natural interventions to help promote a good night's sleep and they are part of the "Sleep Naturally Plan."

Behavior and Thought Change in the Sleep Naturally Plan

To fail to accept that every night will not bring perfect sleep is a major bar to good sleeping. Individuals with a new onset of insomnia must examine their lifestyle and listen to their body. Changes in daily routines, especially exercise and eating, can affect sleep and there are milestones in our life where sleep patterns change. Women around the time of menstruation can sleep less or more; and the menopause (cessation of periods) is often heralded by sleeplessness. Thus, the concept of natural variations in sleep habits must be accepted, unless sleep deprivation is clearly causing impairment of social or physical functions.

Table 9 highlights some thoughts about sleep for the sleepless. These thoughts can result in changes of attitudes or behavior when it comes to sleep. When considering thoughts, attitudes and behavior, one must eliminate the mental "bed of nails." Sleep does not readily occur in a challenging or uncomfortable environment, bedroom or bed.

Thought	Resolution
Many people sleep more than they think they do	Just like obese persons who underestimate their calorie intake, many insomniacs have a very skewed perception of their own sleep patterns. Unpleasant portions of sleep are those that are remembered. A self-analysis of sleep duration and quality is often reassuring.

Sleep analysis?	Some behavioral scientists believe in the value of keeping a sleep log book. This permits an individual to look for cause and effect in sleep disorders. To learn that a cup of coffee or one glass of wine too many inhibits sleep is valuable information for behavior change.
Is my sleep environment -optimal?	Factors as banal as good sleepwear, safe hot water bottles, dim lights or total absence of light in a bedroom can make a real difference.
Bedtime is not the time for the "worry of the day"	"Brain-lock" affects many people. It is normal in the absence of distractions to focus on events that are key issues in one's life. Coping strategies are important and identifying a "worry time" during the middle of the day permits one to shelve worries to a workable schedule that does not rob sleep.
Do not seek comfort in periods of nocturnal wakefulness	Individuals may see their hours of nocturnal insomnia as periods of time to cherish. This may come out of a need to have "private time" away from the "hustle and bustle" of the household. "Private time" must be fitted to a daytime schedule.
Adjustments to poor sleep patterns are necessary	For some, sleep problems just do not go away. Good planning can separate needs to perform from periods of insomnia. Attempts to put off or rearrange activities that require maximum physical and mental functioning can be rewarded with a new sense of well-being.
Avoid the panic of the chronic insomniac	Falling asleep gives rise to a type of early sleep that recharges batteries, but later patterns of sleep are important for mood control and memory. The person who awakes at points in the middle of the night should practice soothing

	acts that can promote and avoid mounting anxiety. Rituals, such as mental imagery, reading or counting blessings, can have a beneficial effect.
Accepting the inevitable disturbances of sleep patterns	Bad news, business reversals and self-remorse are the enemies of sleep, but they do not persist. Men experiencing the change of life (andropause) and women at the time of the menopause start to sleep less. In the elderly, sleep time is often reduced by up to one hour on a nightly basis. This shift of the body's sleep clock is a normal part of aging and is best left untampered.
Sleeping pills and supplements	"Hands down" natural dietary supplements that promote sleep are better than any sleeping drug. Sleeping pills have a well-deserved bad reputation for expense, hangovers and significant other side effects. Allegedly gentler sleeping pills (e.g. Ambien and Sonata). Any sleeping drug can cause dependence (addiction) if taken continuously for longer than a month. Modern science increasingly supports natural agents to support sleep including selected herbs, relaxing minerals and melatonin in a synergistic blend, e.g. Sleep Naturally™, www.sleepnaturally.com. I do not mind being accused of having "my own axe to grind" – natural ways to healthy sleep are to be preferred.

Table 9: Changes in attitudes and behavior that can promote sleep with specific emphasis on a natural approach (www.sleepnaturally.com). This advice is a fundamental component of the "Sleep Naturally Plan."

Sleep Centers

The rapid increases in the number of sleep centers through the country attest to the swelling ranks of Americans seeking help for sleep disorders. Hundreds of independent sleep centers or smaller facilities attached to hospitals have emerged in recent times. While the number of sleep laboratories may not be enough to accommodate millions of patients with sleep disorders, the information they gather from the patients may help provide a better understanding of sleep. This valuable information can guide future research. Sleep has become big business for doctors, clinics and hospitals.

An accredited sleep center is usually run by board-certified physicians specializing in sleep disorders. An individual needing service at a sleep center will have to provide the facility with a medical background and a history of the sleep disorder. While sleep centers are special "laboratories" for sleep disorders, the health care professionals in a sleep center attempt to treat the cause of the sleep disorder, not just the symptoms. Treatment at sleep centers may include medical interventions using prescriptions drugs, sleep devices or behavior modification. Advice to lose weight, quit smoking and avoid excessive alcohol intake is common advice from sleep centers staff. Sleep centers are equipped with a wide range of measurement instruments and various devices to treat sleep problems, such as nasal dilators, dental appliances, airway pressure devices, etc.

The Bed You Lie On

Correct posture is important for general well-being. Medical disciplines, such as Chiropractic medicine and the application of the Alexander technique, focus on the importance of spinal alignment for disease prevention and treatment. During sleep, correct posture helps prevent back aches and overall soreness of the body. Over the years, beds and mattresses have evolved to conform to the individual's sleeping needs. Innovations in mattress or bed designs have resulted in complicated choices for consumers when it comes to bed purchases. Specially designed beds are being promoted actively in the media by manufacturers. It is notable that some bed manufacturers have actually engaged in clinical research to demonstrate the benefits of their various bed designs.

The degree of softness or firmness of mattress plays a major role in the average person's decision to purchase a bed. New technology has provided beds that have sleeping sections that can be varied in their degree of firmness. One such popular bed is called the "Sleep Number Bed". This particular bed has remote controls that permit alteration of the mattress to suit an individual's need. The mattress has a wide range of settings from ultimate softness through to almost rigid flatness. It is notable that this bed has been subjected to research studies in people who have set the mattress "firmness levels" of these beds to their own level of comfort. Such studies are reported to have been performed by researchers at Duke University and UCLA. Simple outcomes of these studies showed quite impressive improvements in the initiation of sleep and staying asleep.

These research studies on the Sleep Number Bed also showed that individuals with simple types of back ache had symptomatic improvements when using the Sleep Number Bed. Principal explanations for these benefits may rest in the knowledge that correct spinal posture is obviously important in the management of backache. Several Chiropractic physicians have endorsed this type of approach to improve sleeping habits. There are other types of mattresses that can adjust to body contours, as a result of their special compression characteristics. One type of bed uses plastics technology to match body contours. This technology was developed by NASA. In addition, there are mechanical beds that can alter body posture during sleep and the "vibrating bed" that can help some people fall asleep.

Sleep Problems at Specific Times of Life

God forbid that any family would be stricken by the tragedy of Sudden Infant Death Syndrome (SIDS). Any abnormality in sleep patterns in babies or infants must be immediately reported to a physician. There has been much research on "cot deaths" and many reasons have been proposed to explain these tragic events. Factors such as exposure of a baby to tobacco smoke during pregnancy or following birth, poor prenatal care or adverse lifestyle in pregnant woman, premature birth, infections and even the act of bottle feeding have all been implicated as potential causes of SIDS.

Over the past decade or so are raging arguments have occurred about the role of body posture in the predisposition of infants to cot deaths. It appears that simple advice on sleeping posture has made a big difference to the occurrence of crib deaths (SIDS). The current recommendation is to have babies sleep on their backs. However, it is only approximately 10 years ago since public agencies and the American Academy of Pediatrics have issued clear directives not to have babies sleep on their stomachs or in a face-down posture.

It is estimated that as many as three-quarters of all newborn infants were placed to sleep in a face-down position in the late 1980s and early 1990s. In several countries where babies are most often put to sleep on their backs, the rate of crib deaths has dropped by a factor of at least 50%. It is striking to note that for almost 50 years of the 20th century many mothers were advised to let their newborns sleep in the face-down or prone position.

While posture is critical for the safety of the newborn, far less attention has been directed to the use of different postures or "posture props" to help adults gain restful sleep. As discussed earlier, high technology beds have been developed, but the strategic use of pillows can certainly benefit the sleepless person. Using a pillow between the legs helps spinal alignment which is not necessarily helped by special mattresses alone. There is some discussion as to whether or not sleeping on one's back or front may have an influence on health. Change in sleep positions seems to be important in young children and studies in Australia have demonstrated that infants who sleep on their backs have less visits to children's outpatient clinics and they may have less problems with coughs, colds and throwing-up after feeding.

Environmental Medicine and Sleep

The "sleeping sleuths" may want to check their sleeping environment for environmental toxins or the quality and comfort of bedding material. Physicians who specialize in environmental medicine have drawn attention to adverse environmental factors in bedrooms and the dietary intake of toxins, such as food colorings, that may contribute to poor sleep. It is known from very careful studies that several aspects of the immune system become primed during sleep and they can be quite reactive. Any allergens in the environment may interact with heightened immunity during sleep and precipitate many disorders. Certainly, attacks of asthma or simple breathing difficulties at night may often have an allergic basis.

Female Hormone Cycles and Sleep

I have discussed the role of biological rhythms in assisting normal sleep patterns and general health. These biological rhythms occur in both men and women but there is no biological rhythm more apparent than the menstrual cycle. Premenstrual disorders such as premenstrual syndrome or premenstrual tension are often associated with disordered sleep. It is known from elegant studies of the hormone profiles of healthy women that sex hormones such as estrogen and progesterone can have a profound effect on the quality and duration of sleep. There is no doubt that hormonal balance can be "out of whack" in many women and this is particularly notable in the perimenopause, at the time of the menopause or for a year or two after the cessation of periods.

Conventional medicine has tended to address this situation by the apparent logical prescription of female hormones, including the contraceptive pill and estrogen supplements or hormone replacement therapy (HRT). Estrogen with or without progesterone has been given at the time of the menopause and for variable periods in the postmenopause. These practices are now questioned as HRT with potent estrogens becomes somewhat questioned in both its medical benefits and adverse effects. Estrogen or hormone replacement therapy with drugs has been associated with several potential serious side effects, such as blood clotting and the promotion of certain types of cancer. These circumstances, together with the common side effects of hormone therapy, such as weight gain and bloating, have caused many females to seek alternatives to conventional types of hormone replacement.

Furthermore, modern research has uncovered other factors, such as insulin resistance and Syndrome X as important to potential causes of irregular menstruation, Polycystic Ovary Syndrome and infertility. Syndrome X is primarily a lifestyle disorder and it is at the basis of many female-specific reproductive problems. In fact, the treatment of PCOS and associated menstrual irregularities is directed at controlling insulin resistance, which is a pivotal factor that causes Syndrome X (obesity, high blood pressure, high blood cholesterol, linked by insulin resistance).

Alternatives to Hormone Replacement Therapies

Several studies in scientific literature have provided evidence that natural phytochemicals (phyto = plant) can play a valuable role in controlling symptoms of premenstrual syndrome (PMS) and adverse symptoms experienced around the menopause. These phytochemicals include a number of herbal or botanical agents that have been shown in independent research to control night sweats in the menopause (hot flashes) and reduce feelings of anxiety. Natural therapies can help balance a woman's hormonal status so that she may be able to relax and sleep. Sleep deprivation is an underestimated component of adverse symptoms and signs that are experienced by a woman with PMS or going through the menopause.

There have been some convincing scientific publications on the value of natural herbal and botanical alternatives for the management of PMS and menopause. In a recent article in Annals of Internal Medicine, a prestigious medical journal, Fredi Kronenberg, Ph.D. and Adriane Fugh-Berman, M.D. have described an evidence-based approach to the use of natural agents found in dietary supplements for the management of PMS and perimenopausal problems. These experts have reviewed many controlled clinical trials which point to the safety and effectiveness of these alternative approaches to adjusting hormone balance in women. This evidence-based approach has been used in the development of a dietary supplement called MenoPlan™ (www.menoplan.com, Holt S, The MenoPlan, Wellness Publishing, Newark, NJ, 2003). Yet again, one can see the close links between sleep science and general well-being.

Electrical and Electromagnetic Stimulation of the Body

There are many different techniques in alternative medicine practice to promote the balance of body functions. One emerging and useful technique is the use of stimulation of the body by low-voltage (small) electric currents or magnetic devices. In the excellent book entitled, "The Healing Nutrients Within," Eric R. Braverman, M.D. and his colleagues described multiple benefits of low-voltage electrical stimulation of the brain, using a technique called "Cranial Electrical Stimulation". This type of therapy has been used to benefit a wide variety of disorders including drug abuse, depression, learning disorders, hyperactivity and insomnia.

There are many reports of the benefits of "Cranial Electrical Stimulation". This technique involves the use of a machine that generates a minute electrical current that is applied as a stimulus to the brain. There are portable devices that deliver Cranial Electrical Stimulation for use at home. Dr. Braverman and his colleagues have published favorable results using Cranial Electrical Stimulation in the management of drug abuse and several different brain disorders.

The basic hypothesis for the use of minute dose electrical stimulation of the brain is the probable correction of abnormal electrical events (electrophysiological abnormalities) that are associated with many different diseases.

Several researchers have proposed that Cranial Electrical Stimulation may be more beneficial with the use of natural agents, such as amino acids, that can work together with electricity in helping to balance chemicals that transmit nervous impulses in the brain. These matters are discussed in detail by Dr. Braverman and his colleagues in the third edition of the new book "The Healing Nutrients Within", Basic Health Publications, Inc., North Bergen, NJ, 2003.

Chapter Summary

It would not be possible to review in any detail the thousands of sleep aids that exist in the market. Ranging from useless to valuable, these aids are used increasingly by up to 100 million Americans who have a need to engage in restful sleep. Pharmaceuticals (drugs) used for sleeping possess many disadvantages and limitations. Natural agents that can assist sleep patterns may provide some alternatives to drugs for sleep induction (www.sleepnaturally.com). The person who is "hooked" on drugs for sleeping should seek medical attention.

There are several healthy keys to a good night's sleep that involve behavioral changes. Fighting insomnia "head on" creates a vicious cycle of self-directed abuse. Behavior change, lifestyle change and some degree of compromise are often necessary for small but valuable improvements in sleep patterns. Many expert centers have arisen as free-standing sleep centers or hospital-based sleep laboratories. In these new centers, individuals with protracted sleep problems may avail themselves of recent advances in the science of sleep.

Chapter 6:

SLEEP NATURALLY: NUTRITIONAL SUPPORT FOR NATURAL SLEEP

Debunking Some Drug Approaches to Sleep

One must conclude that sleep disorders occur for many reasons, including diseases, biochemical disturbances in the body and psychological factors. One of the principal biochemical disorders that may interfere with sleep is caused by the use of drugs used to induce sleep. Many people are seeking natural alternatives to drugs to deal with their insomnia, but arguments still prevail about the effectiveness of herbs, botanicals and nutritional agents for the induction of sleep. These opinions are changing as more research uncovers the ability of natural agents to contribute to restful sleep.

The pivotal question in the selection of any methods to manage insomnia is: "How long has the difficulty with sleep been present?" Insomnia lasting a short time can be managed with behavior therapy and natural agents, but long-standing insomnia is a state that can lead to long-term drug use – a situation best avoided. It is my opinion that natural ways to healthy sleep are always to be preferred.

Diet and Nutrition for Sleep

Diet and general nutrition is a key factor that promotes healthy sleep. Many drugs and alcohol can disturb the sleeping process. Few people realize that heavy drinking can reduce overall sleep time and it seriously impairs the quality of sleep, by altering both REM and non-REM sleep phases. There are many similarities between the effects of alcohol on sex and its effects on sleep. Alcohol can increase the desire for sex or sleep, but it interferes with the performance of these natural acts. Caffeine is ubiquitous in the American diet and it has a common and profound effect on sleeping habits. The sensitivity of an individual to the stimulatory effects of caffeine varies greatly from person to person.

Not only has excessive caffeine consumption been associated with poor sleep, it contributes to disorders such as "restless leg syndrome" and periodic body movements that can interrupt sleep. In addition, caffeine can have significant effects on the rapidity and rhythm of heartbeats. Caffeine finds its way into many foods and beverages, e.g. cola, several carbonated beverages, cough and cold remedies. Caffeine is a principal component of "alleged" weight-reducing, natural products (natural slimming capsules), most of which are of dubious benefit. Even a couple of cups of coffee or caffeine containing tea, on a daily basis, can interfere with both the quality and quantity of sleep.

Food Intolerance and Insomnia

Some physicians have suggested that food intolerance, or "food allergies," may contribute to poor sleep. Foods implicated as a potential cause of insomnia include cereal grains (wheat and corn), dairy produce and chocolate. A warm glass of milk at night is a soothing preparation for many people at their bedtime, but in some people with milk intolerance it may cause wakefulness.

The role of food intolerance in causing stress, tension, anxiety or wakefulness is not well defined in conventional medicine. Experts in food intolerance or allergy emphasize that susceptible individuals may be troubled by inability to concentrate and even major degrees of restlessness during the day. It may be that people suffering from food intolerance exhibit greater than normal irritability during waking hours. Whether or not this form of food intolerance produces changes in body chemistry that provoke wakefulness remains an underexplored area, but food exclusion diets may be helpful for promoting sleep in selected people.

Attention to the Sleep Environment

Several immediate factors in the sleep environment have been alleged to cause insomnia. British researchers have drawn attention to the generation of unwanted electric or magnetic fields by a variety of sleep aids. Certainly, electromagnetic fields are created by heated beds, blankets, stereo systems and computers that sometimes clutter a bedroom. There are obvious changes one can make to a bedroom that will help encourage restful sleep. These include good control of environmental temperature, humidity, noise, etc.

Overuse of Sleep Medications: Real Dangers of OTC Hypnotic Drugs

There are about 10 million Americans that fill prescriptions for sleeping drugs and millions of people who buy over-the-counter (OTC) hypnotic drugs (antihistamines). It has been argued that this pattern of drug use has resulted in a major change in sleep patterns in many people. Drugs to induce sleep characteristically lose their effectiveness over a period of two or three months and some sleeping tablets commonly cause a morning hangover, residual drowsiness and poor physical or mental performance. All hypnotic drugs interact with alcohol in an addictive and negative manner.

A major concern is the potential development of addiction and withdrawal symptoms with drugs for sleep induction. Indeed, sleep patterns can be worse after periods of treatment with sleeping drugs. The use of over-the-counter drugs to sleep is not universally safe. These drugs often belong to a class of drugs called antihistamines. These antihistamines can accumulate in the body and they are often "long-acting." The use of OTC drugs for sleep can cause delirium, especially in the elderly. Delirium is a severe form of a confusional state.

The class of drugs called antihistamines is the active component in almost all OTC hypnotic drugs. As previously mentioned, these drugs block histamine receptors and have their primary use in the treatment of allergies, not sleep disorders. Antihistamine drugs interfere with parts of the nervous system that are composed of cholinergic nerves. This cholinergic nervous system is responsible for regulating bowel action, bladder function, blood pressure, vision and the secretion of fluids that cover mucous membranes, such as the mouth and nasal passages.

Antihistamine drugs have quite strong antagonistic actions on the cholinergic nervous system, i.e. they are anti-cholinergic. These actions of OTC hypnotic drugs often cause a dry mouth, blurred vision and hangover effect, such as "grogginess" and even confusion immediately after waking. People with high pressure in their eyes (glaucoma), any form of dementia (e.g. Alzheimer's disease) and enlargement of the prostate should avoid OTC drugs that contain antihistamines.

It should be noted that many common cough and cold remedies contain sedating antihistamines to deal with the symptoms of flu. These popular cough and cold remedies share the same side effects as OTC drugs used for sleep. In addition, these anti-cholinergic effects can result in constipation, retention of urine and lowering of blood pressure inappropriately when people stand up quickly or get out of bed quickly (orthostatic hypotension).

Unexpected falls in blood pressure when getting out of bed is a very serious problem in mature individuals or the elderly. Unexpected falls in blood pressure can cause dizziness, loss of balance and it is an important factor in accidents and falls in the elderly. Mature and elderly people may have thin bones (osteoporosis) and these individuals are particularly susceptible to bone fractures such as hip fractures, spinal fractures and wrist fractures. I have discussed the important public health concerns that exist in the prevention and management of osteoporosis in the elderly in my book entitled "The Antiporosis Plan".

Information about accidents in the elderly and education to avoid such accidents is very important in any account of sleep and its disorders. Falls at home and hip fractures in the elderly can compromise the quality of life in the elderly, result in institutionalization and sometimes cause death in the short to intermediate term following injury. Therefore, the safety of OTC sleep drugs must be reappraised and my advice is that they be avoided completely, because of their onerous side effect profile.

Dietary Supplements May Have Real Advantages

I stress that dietary supplements containing natural agents have undergone very few scientific comparisons with hypnotic drugs and the kind of controlled research that has occurred with some pharmaceuticals may far outweigh scientific studies of natural sleeping agents. However, the science behind the use of nutritional or herbal agents to support sleep has strengthened dramatically over the past 10 years, especially in relationship to our knowledge about the ability of natural hormones to help sleep, e.g. melatonin and botanicals, e.g. Valerian. Furthermore, certain herbs to assist sleep have been used for more than a thousand years with safety and effectiveness, e.g. Valerian.

I stress that many natural agents have a very long precedent of effectiveness and a history of repeated use with a high margin of safety. I do not believe that any agent, drug, or otherwise, used to support sleep should be used in isolation of behavioral treatment. These behavioral treatments include but are not limited to: behavioral change, well planned exercise, avoidance of substance abuse, meditation, massage and breathing exercises, etc. One particularly attractive area of "alternative" management of insomnia is the use of bio-feedback treatment. In bio-feedback treatments, health care givers can monitor body functions, such as anxiety, and give positive reinforcement by counseling or simple relaxation exercise. Relaxation responses to anything are valuable in sleep promotion, e.g. listening to music, reading, etc.

A Multi-Pronged Approach to Sleeping: No "Magic Bullets"

It is clear that the approach to insomnia must be a multi-pronged approach and a very careful patient history is often the best way of identifying some of the many factors that may interfere with restful sleep (Table 10). The questions in Table 10 are what a doctor may ask a patient about sleep problems. I am convinced that the first-line option to sleep disorders must be a combination of simple, gentle, natural approaches. These approaches include detailed attention to good lifestyle and the potential use of natural agents that may help promote sleep in a safe and effective manner (Sleep Naturally™, www.sleepnaturally.com).

Natural ways to healthy sleep may be exercised before the use of potent sleeping drugs or other pharmaceuticals which carry disadvantages or limitations in their application. Drugs to promote sleep have problems, including cost and unwanted side effects, as part of an unfortunate drug "band aid approach" to insomnia. There must be a widespread realization that our current level of scientific knowledge has not provided us with a "magic bullet" to correct sleep problems. Sleep has so many controlling factors that no single agent can be expected to be universally successful for sleep problems

- The duration of sleep problems is a critical question. Chronic insomnia spells trouble
- Careful questions about medications, use of illicit drugs and substance abuse, including caffeine, alcohol and tobacco. Questions should focus on existing use of sleep medication, any mood changes, behavioral problems or psychiatric disease
- The following sleep characteristics must be defined: "normal" sleep, pattern, type of sleep disturbance, functioning in the daytime, assessment of sleep cycles (24-hour, Circadian Rhythm) and clinical course of the sleep disorders
- Any past or family history of sleep problems (narcolepsy is often hereditary)
- Onset, frequency, severity, precipitation, relieving factors for sleep problems
- Information from bed partner can be extremely important in diagnosis

Table 10: The content of questions that a doctor or health care-giver may ask about sleeping, in order to make a diagnosis, select a treatment or order medical testing.

Developing an Optimal, Natural Dietary Supplement to Support Sleep

Seldom in my writings have I related personal experience. Any such experience must be biased. As a member of the medical profession, I am no stranger to forced periods of sleeplessness and less of a stranger to stress that has interfered with my own sleep patterns. My family members and I have made many common errors in our attempts to gain restful sleep. Fortunately, I have not suffered from significant, chronic insomnia, but more than my fair share of sleepless nights compelled me to research various natural ways to engage the act of restful sleep. Over a period of approximately 10 years, I have taken all natural agents for which there is reasonable, good scientific agreement for a benefit in sleep assistance; and I have used them in varying combinations in order to seek an optimal combination of natural substances to promote sleep.

My personal research is not more than empiric, but who questioned the value of serendipity?

The Concept of Synergy in Natural Dietary Supplement Formulations

It has become increasingly apparent to me that several natural substances known to assist in the induction or prolongation of sleep are best used in safe, low dosage combinations. For example, melatonin is a natural agent that I have researched extensively. Although I can state with confidence that melatonin is effective in many people when used alone, there is an inevitable requirement for people to increase the dosage of melatonin from about one or two milligrams up to as much as nine or ten milligrams, if they wish to sustain the beneficial sleep-inducing effects of this natural hormone. This raises a major problem. While small milligram doses of melatonin are safe, I cannot attest to the safety of higher doses of melatonin, the use of which must be supervised by the close attention of a skilled medical practitioner.

What comes out of my line of reasoning is that small doses of a number of safe agents that promote sleep can all act together to be more effective than when they are used in isolation. This is the concept of "synergy," where each relatively small dose of a natural substance that promotes sleep works together, in concert, to produce a superior overall effect. Synergy is now emerging in leading-edge nutraceutical technology as the "way to go." There is another, underestimated benefit to the use of smaller doses of natural substances that have a "helper" effect on each other (a synergistic effect). This benefit is the tendency of "the mix" to avoid the development of tolerance to the ingredients. Rapid tolerance can develop to single agents, including natural agents or single drugs. When "tolerance" develops, the single agent becomes ineffective; and more has to be used with the greater possibility of toxicity. A complex array of "helper substances" can help avoid tolerance or the "wearing off" of the sleep inducing effects of natural substances.

The Sleep Naturally Formula

A reasonably optimal combination of natural agents for sleep that I have combined with synergistic effects, is prominently stated below:

Sleep Naturally™ is nutritional support for the body function of sleep.

SUPPLEMENT FACTS: Servings per container: 30 Serving Size 2 Capsules Contain

Ingredients Amount A Proprietary Blend of Valerian Root, Chamomile Flower, Passionflower, Lemon Balm, Skullcap Whole, Hops Whole and Ashwagandha Root 650 mg 5 Hydroxytryptophan (5HTP) 10 mg Magnesium (Oxide) (50% RDI) 200 mg Melatonin 2 mg Niacin (50% RDI) 10 mg Vitamin B6 (Pyridoxine HCL) (100% RDI) 2 mg Folic Acid (100% RDI) 0.4 mg

Warning: For adult use only at bedtime. This product is not to be taken by pregnant or lactating women. If you are taking medication or have a medical condition, consult a physician before using this product. Do not use in conjunction with alcoholic beverages, when driving a vehicle or while operating machinery. Natural substances may interfere with drug treatments and vice versa. All potential drug or disease interactions should be discussed with a medical practitioner.

There are many different dietary supplements that claim to provide nutritional support for sleep and some go as far as making the "unregulated claim" of being a "sleeping tablet." It must be emphasized that dietary supplements cannot be used to diagnose, prevent or cure any disease; and it is important that people understand that they can sometimes mask serious diseases that contribute to or compound sleep problems, by taking many drugs or dietary supplements.

Avoid Interactions Between Drugs, Diseases and Dietary Supplements

In cases of doubt about sleeping aids, readers are referred to qualified physicians. Anyone taking medications must make sure that there is no possibility of drug interaction. The real use of Sleep Naturally™ and other dietary supplements is in people with simple sleep problems.

Self-medication in the presence of significant illness is not advised. The evidence to support the inclusion of various natural substances in the Sleep Naturally Plan™ should be studied by the user; and I encourage dialogue between physicians and patients and vice versa. I am somewhat surprised that many people will use dietary supplements without obtaining education in their safe use. Please enjoy the information provided in this chapter of the book, but use it safely!

Valerian (Valeriana officinalis)

Valerian root is a pungent herb with an unpleasant smell. Herbalists have used Valerian extensively as a minor sedative and it is useful for managing states of excitation, nervous anxiety and insomnia. It assists the body in general relaxation and it is quite valuable as a sedative in the presence of stress, discomfort or pain.

On a practical basis, Valerian is very useful for minor sedation. In addition to this sedative action, Valerian root has well-described anticonvulsant activity, meaning that it acts against epilepsy or seizures. Valerian is quite useful in people with jerks during sleep (myoclonus) and in some people with the "restless leg syndrome." Valerian depresses the nervous system in a gentle manner at moderate doses and it may help prevent seizures, but it is not a reliable treatment for seizure disorders. Careful scientific studies show that Valerian interferes with the function of certain molecules that pass messages in the brain and nervous system. It inhibits the enzymatic breakdown of the neurotransmitter gamma-amino-butyric acid, GABA.

Valerian used in Sleep Naturally™ comes from the underground parts (rhizome and roots) of the plant Valeriana officinalis. Valerian has been widely used in Europe for its digestive benefits (carminative) and calming effects. It is notable that Valerian root has more than one thousand years of history of use for its sedating effects. Few beneficial "treatment" agents survive throughout a period of a millennium without consistency of experienced benefits.

Valerian has a long tradition of use as a sedative known to relieve conditions of insomnia, anxiety, fatigue, migraine, etc. and it has been used often as a mild form of tranquilizer. Clinical studies have shown that extracts of Valerian root administered to insomniacs have resulted in better sleep for the subjects.

The sedative properties of Valerian have been compared with those of barbiturates and benzodiazepines. In these comparisons, Valerian herb did not result in significant hangover effects of morning sleepiness in people who used it, compared with certain benzodiazepine or barbiturate drugs. Valerian is known to exert maximum benefits when the body is free of caffeine, alcohol and other unwanted substances. The U.S. Food and Drug Administration has declared the Valerian plant to be safe when used appropriately, paving the way for its use in nutritional supplements where "calming effects" are required (www.sleepnaturally.com).

Valerian Root: Adaptogenic and Synergistic

The active constituents of Valerian remain unclear. Constituents of Valerian root called valpotriates act as muscle relaxants, such that they have a special role in relieving muscle spasms. Recently, water extracts of Valerian, containing the ingredient valeric acid, have been shown to have significant sedative actions. Thus, there is more than one chemical in Valerian root that may act together (synergistically) to account for its well defined, beneficial actions.

On the one hand, Valerian can calm the agitated person, whereas on the other, Valerian can be a mild stimulant in cases of fatigue. This "balancing" effect of this herb is called an "adaptogenic effect." An "adaptogen" is a safe substance that has a balancing effect on body functions and increases the body's resistance to stress. It is notable that several natural substances are adaptogens (balancing agents). Adaptogenic herbs are a great secret of "Nature" and it makes natural agents to promote sleep desirable.

Other Benefits of Valerian

Valerian has some extra benefits for health that are not as well known as its hypnotic or calming actions. Some studies show that Valerian may assist in lowering elevated blood pressure, increasing the flow of bile from the liver (a choleretic effect), anti-cancer effects, some antibiotic activity and an ability to relieve colic or muscle spasms in the intestines. How does Valerian work?

Recent studies have shown that extracts of Valerian (valeric acid and valpotriates) are able to act like benzodiazepine drugs. These compounds (extracts of Valerian) work on the same receptors in the brain as drugs like Valium® (benzodiazepines). However, Valium® has side effects of causing confusion and impairing mental function, whereas Valerian does not tend to cause these problems. Furthermore, Valerian does not cause a "hangover" or addiction (dependency) like the drug Valium®. Several physicians have commented on the ability of the Valerian to be switched for benzodiazepine drugs, for obvious reasons. However, this switch should be medically supervised. Perhaps Mother Nature knows best!

Chamomile (Matricara recutita)

Chamomile can provide versatile, calming comfort. It has been used for several centuries both internally for its multiple potential benefits and on the skin as a healing agent for rashes and itching problems. Chamomile preparations are made from the flowers of a small "daisy" found mainly in Germany and Italy. Preparations of chamomile are regarded as quite safe and they have even been used in childhood and pregnancy with apparent safety. However, as with all herbals and botanicals, rare skin rashes occur in people with allergy problems. Table 11 describes the striking, potential healing actions of Chamomile.

Reduces inflammation	Helps ear aches
Improves cough and cold symptoms	Calms nerves
Reduces menstrual cramps	Soothes toothache
Digestive benefits	Relieves skin rashes
May prevent peptic ulcers	Assists sleep
Relieves gum disease and oral irritation	Relaxes the stomach and intestines

Table 11: Potential benefits of Chamomile that have been mentioned in scientific and folklore, herbal writings

Chamomile: A Clever Bag of Tricks

Chamomile contains various natural compounds that work together to provide a health benefit. These compounds have been studied in oils distilled from chamomile flower heads. They include chamazulene, bisabolol and a variety of bioflavonoids that have antioxidant actions. The flavonoids include substances, such as apigenin and luteolin. Chamomile is a true mixed bag of "magical, natural tricks" and this accounts for its widespread popularity in Western Europe.

A common reason for sleeplessness in many people is a "heavy" late night meal. While best avoided, social occasions often present this circumstance. Chamomile is particularly good at relaxing a full stomach. It has a carminative (digestive) effect with the added benefit of mild sedation. Chamomile has been grossly underestimated as a versatile, soothing herb in American medical practice.

Chamomile Cuts "Cramps"

Chamomile has been widely used as a mild sedative and it has smooth muscle relaxing activity. Smooth muscles found in the organs of the digestive tract can go into spasm and cause "cramps" or colic. Chamomile has been described as particularly valuable for digestive upset associated with "spasm" that occurs with nervousness, stress and excitement. Chamomile is a complex mixture of bioactive compounds, many of which function as "antispasmodics" (relieve colic or spasm in the gut). It is a tried and trusted remedy for anxiety and its related behavioral associations. Chamomile has also gained recognition for its benefits as a topical agent for eczema and psoriasis. Chamomile is a general purpose, safe and versatile herb that can assist in managing an individual's behavioral problems.

Ashwagandha (Withania somnifera)

Ashwagandha is an herb with a long-standing use in Ayurvedic medicine, where it is used as a general "nerve" tonic. The discipline of Ayurvedic medicine is one of the most ancient forms of traditional medicine, developed more than two thousand years ago. It is very interesting to note the word Ashwagandha means "vitality of the horse" in ancient Sanskrit language. The root of the plant is used and it is sometimes called "winter cherry". The plant grows at elevated positions of about 6000 feet, especially in the Himalayan Mountains.

Ashwagandha has been used most often as an "adaptogenic" herb (balancing) with general tonic actions. It is believed to be particularly valuable in the elderly and in animals when general debility is present. Its general benefits are best understood by the reference to Ashwagandha as the example of "Indian Ginseng".

There have been many studies of the use of Ashwagandha root in Ayurvedic healing and it is becoming increasingly popular in North America. To summarize its actions, Ashwagandha is referred to in Ayurvedic medicine as a nervine (compare with skullcap), an astringent, a rejuvenating herb, a sedative, a tonic and an aphrodisiac. "Nervines" are herbs that support the functions of the central nervous system and nerve tissues in general. They have anti-stress actions. Ashwagandha is an herb that helps to build several body functions in states of nervous debility, while allaying anxiety by its mild sedative actions.

Passionflower (Passiflora incarnata)

Passionflower extracts have enjoyed most use as a minor tranquilizer and they have been used extensively in folklore medicine as a female tonic. Preparations of Passionflower are made from the flowers, leaves and fruit of the creeping vine (Passiflora incarnata). The real use of Passionflower is as an adaptogen or a substance that helps "balance" the body, especially in terms of the function of the nervous system. Passionflower can be used in females to calm the mind that may be disturbed by periods of repeated hormonal adjustments. Although Passionflower has been recognized as being of particular value in females, it exerts useful calming effects in males.

Passionflower is regarded as an effective remedy for nerves that are on edge. J. Lutomski, M.D., has drawn attention to the balance brought to the female body by Passionflower in the article entitled: Die Bedeutung der Passionsblume in der Heilkunde, published in the journal, Pharmazie in unserer Zeit, in 1981 (10,2, pp.45-49). Roughly translated, the title of this paper is “The Meaning of Passionflower in Current Times.” The tranquilizing benefits of passionflower are particularly useful in nervous manifestations of menstrual problems and menopause. According to Dr. Varro Tyler in his famous book “Herbs of Choice,” there are no known side effects or contraindications to Passionflower.

Lemon Balm (Melissa officinalis)

Lemon balm is derived from a plant that grows mainly in the Eastern Mediterranean and the Western parts of Asia. It contains a number of essential oils and polyphenolic compounds. Its effects are wide-ranging and very interesting. The common form of lemon balm is a sedative with antispasmodic actions. In naturopathic medicine, it is highly regarded as an antibacterial agent. It has been employed most often for gastrointestinal and cardiovascular disorders that are “nervous” in origin. It is a classic “nervine”. Experiments in mice have shown lemon balm to have both sedative and pain-killing effects.

Extensive accounts of its use in folklore medicine describe its calming ability without the occurrence of a “hangover”. It has been regarded as particularly valuable in states of melancholia (sadness) and hysteria (extreme agitation). This makes lemon balm very valuable for the nervous or dependent individual. Lemon balm has been reported to be effective in reversing rapid heart beats (palpitations) that are precipitated by nervousness. While lemon balm is calming, it is also described as a “strengthening” remedy. It has an interesting ability to correct nervous disorders that interfere with sleep; and it can correct anxiety-induced effects on the gastrointestinal tract. In circumstances of debility, lemon balm has been useful at stimulating appetite. Lemon balm is regarded as quite safe and particularly valuable in circumstances of anxiety, “jitters” while under stress and excitement induced by changes in the environment.

Catnip (Nepeta cateria)

Catnip is an intriguing herb that acts generally as a mild tranquilizer or sedative that allays anxiety and helps promote restful sleep. When catnip is taken orally, it does not tend to cause euphoria in the same way that occurs as a consequence of "sniffing" the herb, especially in cats. Catnip has a special role in settling the stomach and bowels of individuals. As mentioned, some individuals respond with digestive upset (diarrhea or vomiting) to stress in their environment and for them catnip can work "like a charm."

Skullcap (Scutellaria laterifolia)

Skullcap belongs to the "mint" family of plants and it has sedative, anxiolytic and anticonvulsant properties. It is referred to by herbalists as a "nervine" because of its special actions on the nervous system. For many years, Skullcap has been used to treat acute and chronic nervous disorders, where anxiety predominates.

Skullcap seems to have versatile actions on the nervous system. It calms "jittery nerves", but it does not cause drowsiness. The herb has been called an "adaptogen" because of its ability to calm or balance nervous behavior in certain individuals, without inducing sleep. During times of rehabilitation from injury, Skullcap appears to have special value. It has a calming effect but does not dull the senses. Skullcap is not advised for use in pregnancy, while breastfeeding, or in the presence of significant liver disease.

Hops (Humulus lupulus)

Hops are best known for their bitter taste which is used in the brewing of beer. The oxidation of the bitter principle of Hops, called humulene, gives beers a typical flavor. The late Dr. Varro E. Tyler, Ph.D. notes that people who picked hops became easily tired because they were exposed to resin from hop plants which may have acted as a sedative.

This plant contains many different, potentially active ingredients. Many belong to a class of compounds called polyphenols. Polyphenols are antioxidant compounds. Animal experiments have shown that hops possess both sedative and sleep-inducing properties. One type of alcohol found in hops may account for the sedative properties. Extracts of hops are known to inhibit or smooth muscle contraction and this has led to the use of this herb as an antispasmodic for intestinal colic.

There is considerable debate about the active principle that may be present in hops, but it is clear that hops should be used when fresh, because this herb can rapidly lose its potency. The potentially active compounds in hops include humulone (humulene), lupulone, myrcene and other resinous compounds. It is of interest that hops are "close cousins" of marijuana, but hops do not seem to induce the same effects as cannabis.

5-Hydroxytryptophan (5-HTP)

5-hydroxytryptophan has been used for a variety of indications in alternative medicine. It seems to exert benefit in individuals with fibromyalgia and anxiety disorders, but its principal use has been as a sedative and potential sleep aid. 5-HTP has been studied in people with depression and found to exert several benefits. Other described benefits of 5-HTP include positive actions in some degenerative nervous system diseases and weight loss. Some of the actions of 5-HTP on several diseases are quite variable in positive outcomes.

The precursor molecule to 5-HTP is L-tryptophan. L-tryptophan is an amino acid that has been associated with serious blood and muscle disorders, due to its contamination with certain chemicals. This contamination gave L-tryptophan a bad name, but L-tryptophan is found in food. Most scientists agree that in the absence of contamination, L-tryptophan is safe. Because of the development of problems with L-tryptophan, 5-HTP has become quite popular as an alternative. Only 5-HTP that has no chance of being contaminated must be used. The common side effects of 5-HTP in large doses include gastrointestinal disturbances, but 5-HTP is used in a small, safe, synergistic dosage in Sleep Naturally™.

Melatonin

The natural hormone melatonin is a master controller of the onset of sleep and other biological functions of the body that repeat themselves on a daily basis. In other words, melatonin controls several "Circadian Activities." A small portion of the front of the brain called the hypothalamus is responsible for controlling the secretion of melatonin by the pineal gland. The pineal gland is located deep in the back of the brain.

Cycles of secretion of melatonin occur with a specific rhythm that is controlled by exposure to light and dark in the environment. Melatonin is very necessary for good sleep and its secretion in the body is subdued to a major degree by exposure to bright light. In fact, it is known that the length of time that melatonin is secreted by the pineal gland is closely related to duration of the night or dark environments. In simple terms, melatonin is responsible for telling the body what to do in response to cycles of daylight and darkness. Melatonin plays a role in changing body functions and general behavior at different times in a daily cycle.

Melatonin has emerged as a safe and effective natural aid for sleep and relaxation. It is particularly effective in people who lose normal patterns of light and dark exposure in their life. Much benefit from the use of melatonin can be achieved by travelers or shift workers who keep irregular hours. Not only can melatonin help in putting people to sleep in a natural way, it can also help to sustain sleep, without producing a morning hangover. Melatonin has shown benefits in helping people withdraw from certain types of sleeping pills (benzodiazepines), but medical supervision is required for this kind of "switching."

Melatonin has been described as having many different benefits, including potential anti-cancer effects, stimulation of immune function, improvement in mood in selected people and specific roles in promoting women's health (combat against osteoporosis and PMS). Melatonin has been described as one of the major anti-stress defenses of the body and it has had special applications in the treatment of jet lag. More recently, several studies have claimed the benefit of melatonin as an anti-aging hormone. A condition called "the Melatonin Deficiency Syndrome" has been proposed, because levels of melatonin do fall with age. Melatonin is a powerful antioxidant and it plays a major role in diminishing oxidative stress that causes tissue aging and the development of a variety of chronic diseases.

Melatonin is well tolerated by most people and it has a low occurrence of side effects. Even very large amounts of melatonin do not cause death in experimental animals. High doses of melatonin have been associated with some side effects, including gastrointestinal upset, headaches and flushing. Melatonin should be avoided in pregnancy, childhood and during breastfeeding. While some animal studies suggested suppression of hormone responses from the pituitary gland with melatonic administration, this phenomenon does not apparently occur in humans.

Some scientists have argued that melatonin may cause certain autoimmune conditions and any use of melatonin in people with autoimmune disorders should occur under medical supervision. While melatonin has a low occurrence of side effects, I do not believe that it is safe in high dosage when taken over very prolonged periods of time. I have limited the amount of melatonin in the product Sleep Naturally™ to a dosage of 2 mg daily. This desirable but effective amount of melatonin forms an important part of the empiric synergy found in the dietary supplement Sleep Naturally™. (www.sleepnaturally.com). One word of caution is important: The use of melatonin in serious psychiatric disorders should be closely monitored.

The ability of melatonin to help reset biological rhythms is very valuable in the treatment of jet lag and people with difficulty in falling asleep. I find it surprising that melatonin is not recommended more often by some sleep experts who argue that exposure to bright light in the morning is more effective than melatonin administration at night in resetting biological rhythms. However, much evidence has accumulated that melatonin administration is a safe and healthy way to promote restful sleep. Sleep experts who have dismissed the benefits of melatonin for sleep should take some time to recognize the other, wide-ranging benefits of melatonin administration.

A Serious Look at Odd Hypnotic Drugs

I have been surprised on occasion to find some people with chronic insomnia using obsolete and dangerous sleeping tablets, such as long-acting barbiturates, glutethimide and methyprylon. These drug selections are truly the option of the almost destitute because these drugs have serious side effects and a toxic dose of these drugs is not much greater than the dose of these drugs required to induce sleep. I raise this issue, at this stage, to reinforce the idea that taking a few paces backwards and reexamining natural options for sleep may be more valuable than hitherto supposed by the modern medical community.

Magnesium

Magnesium could easily be described as a relaxing element. Magnesium deficiency is more common generally suspected. Magnesium deficiencies are common in the elderly, as a consequence of stress and even as a result of high protein and high sugar intake in the diet. Lack of magnesium causes symptoms and signs, such as weakness, irritability, nervousness and muscle cramps. Inadequate intake of magnesium or excessive excretion of magnesium by the body can contribute to cardiac disease, abnormal heart rhythms, high blood pressure, resistance to the hormone insulin, thin bones (osteoporosis), migraine, PMS and poor ability to perform exercise.

Most people are aware of the relaxing effects of magnesium and visiting a spa and "drinking the waters" usually amounts to improving magnesium and other mineral intake. Modern research has confirmed the relaxing effects of magnesium where brain wave patterns change to types of activity associated with relaxation responses when magnesium is administered.

Given the wide-ranging potential benefits of magnesium supplementation in the diet, 50% of the recommended daily intake of magnesium at night is an important synergistic component of Sleep Naturally™. There are few circumstances in which magnesium is toxic. These include excessive dosing, especially if an individual has severe kidney disease. Magnesium is clearly a safe, relaxing element and it is about 50% absorbed by most people when taken as a supplement.

Niacin, Vitamin B6 and Folic Acid

Niacin has been promoted as vitamin that is very important in the prevention and management of mental disease, high blood cholesterol, digestive upset, diabetes mellitus and skin disease. It belongs to a class of vitamins called the B vitamins. It is a cousin of vitamin B6 and folic acid that are also present with niacin in the supplement Sleep Naturally™. Vitamins of the B class are very much involved in the making of chemicals in the body that transmit signals in nervous tissue (neurotransmitters, e.g. serotonin). Deficiencies of B vitamins have been associated with insomnia and there is no doubt that increasing the intake of B vitamins is quite effective in helping sleep, especially when these vitamins may be deficient in the diet.

I have included B vitamins as an important additive benefit in the formulation of Sleep Naturally™ . There is a common disorder of high blood homocysteine levels that has been associated with a variety of diseases, including heart attack, angina, ischemic heart disease, osteoporosis and other chronic degenerative disorders. Evidence from the famous "Nurses Nutrition Studies" has shown the benefits of keeping blood homocysteine under control. Many other studies point to health problems with raised blood homocysteine levels. Vitamin B6 and folic acid help to control raised levels of homocysteine in the blood. This is one of several added benefits of certain components of Sleep Naturally™.

Added Benefits of Sleep Naturally™: A Dietary Supplement

Throughout this chapter, I have hinted that many natural substances that are used to promote sleep have other beneficial effects on health. Herbal and botanical agents with sleep-inducing qualities are sources of antioxidants that can reduce oxidative stress to the body. Normal body functions can produce damaging forms of molecules (chemicals) called "free radicals". For example, many free radicals are generated during rigorous exercise and oxidative stress occurs to many body tissues. Free radicals are also present in the environment in the form of chemicals in food, cigarette smoke and other environmental pollutants. Oxidative stress to the body has been associated with the development of many chronic diseases and premature aging. Antioxidants in the dietary supplement Sleep Naturally™ can help reverse oxidative stress. A particularly powerful antioxidant in Sleep Naturally™ is the natural hormone melatonin.

I have discussed the advantages of keeping blood homocysteine levels in check with certain B vitamins and this approach is combined in Sleep Naturally™. The product Sleep Naturally™ contains several natural substances that have "adaptogenic" or balancing effects on body functions. These added benefits of natural substances to promote sleep are not found in any drugs or pharmaceuticals that are used for their hypnotic qualities.

Chapter Summary

It has become clear that combining a number of natural substances that can help promote sleep is advantageous. This approach can be quite safe and effective in assisting people with simple sleep problems. Temporary insomnia is an ideal disorder in which lifestyle change, behavior modification and the help of natural nutritional support for sleep can be quite valuable (www.sleepnaturally.com). About one half of all cases of insomnia are related to anxiety, stress or other psychological problems.

I believe that the problems that have emerged with the long-term use of prescription drugs or over-the-counter drugs for sleeping should make people more aware of alternatives that could form safe, first-line options. The primary approach should always be a behavioral approach, but for the 100 million Americans who cannot sleep well, nutritional support for sleep presents a very attractive option. I encourage people to talk to their health care givers about natural options to gain restful sleep and supervised attempts to "wean off" hypnotic drugs.

Chapter 7:

THE SLEEP NATURALLY PLAN

Pulling It All Together

Difficulty in falling asleep and staying asleep affects at least 30 million Americans on a long-standing basis (chronic insomnia). More than half of the entire American population experience significant insomnia at one time or another. To get a good night's sleep without resorting to drugs or medications is a potential triumph for millions of Americans. While sleep times tend to decrease in the elderly, there is no substantial evidence that this normal reduction in sleep time can cause significant illness.

Anyone attempting to correct their perceived abnormalities in sleeping patterns must seek a correct diagnosis, especially if their sleep problems are severe and long-standing. I have discussed the evaluation of poor sleep in Chapter 1 and Chapter 7, both from the perspectives of self assessment and the type of evaluation that a health care practitioner may make for a person with sleep disorders. Serious sleep disorders should not be "self-medicated" with drugs or natural products. Furthermore, I do not recommend the use of "sleeping" potions in young children, pregnant or nursing females and in anyone who will not use such potions in a responsible manner. Hypnotic drugs prescribed or purchased over-the-counter can be quite dangerous in the hands of depressed people or children.

I would like to make it crystal-clear that natural ways to improve sleep start with simple changes in lifestyle. Any change in lifestyle from adverse to positive must benefit the sleepless person. Modification of behavior and the application of techniques that permit relaxation are extremely valuable. These natural ways to improve sleep must take precedence. In Table 12, I reiterate simple advice for "would-be sleepers".

- If sleep problems are long-standing, medical consultation is required.
- Abnormal sleep patterns or events, such as sleepwalking, narcolepsy and sleep apnea, are not conditions that should be self-managed.
- Individuals must adopt a regular sleep schedule. There are some new techniques that involve certain degrees of deprivation of time spent in bed that can be valuable for insomniacs.
- Everyone who cannot take sleep for granted must engage in regular bedtime routines. Setting the mood for sleep is all important.
- Restful sleep only occurs in the correct environment. Comfort, noise elimination and any gadget that works, such as a sleeping mask, is worth a try.
- The importance of posture during sleep has been grossly underestimated in conventional medicine. The clever use of pillows to support various parts of the trunk or lower limbs can be quite valuable. New types of beds can be adjusted to help the adoption of optimal postures during sleep.
- Idle people cannot sleep. Regular exercise at the right time of the day and attempts to reduce stress benefit sleep patterns.
- Many drugs interfere with sleep and many substances taken in an average American diet can cause wakefulness.
- Alcohol, caffeine, smoking, illicit drug use, diet pills, natural weight control supplements and water pills are enemies of restful sleep. Caffeine comes in some foods, e.g. chocolate.
- If extra help is required with sleeping, one may consider nutritional support to assist and promote sleep.

Table 12: The author's opinions on optimal pathways to improve simple sleep problems.

Specific Techniques to Allay Anxiety and Promote Sleep

The individual with significant insomnia may lie in bed with stubborn persistence. This circumstance can result in occasional dozing, repeated awakenings and a circumstance of self-persecution. Investing 12 hours in bed rest for a couple of hours of sleep is quite unsatisfactory. Behavioral scientists have suggested a technique called "sleep restriction," but this is better called "bed restriction."

Dr. Arthur Spielman of New York is the originator of a technique where people who do not feel sleepy are not encouraged to go to bed or stay in bed. Some individuals with insomnia are advised, on occasion, to experiment with different bed times that fit their own natural sleep cycles. The "Spielman Technique" can be quite useful in cases of chronic insomnia. An individual who can only sleep for 4 hours is encouraged to spend only 4 hours in bed. This means that the persons with insomnia may go to bed much later than normal. This technique does not allow daytime sleeping or "naps." If the new regimented bed restriction results in improvement in the quality of sleep, the time spent in bed can be extended until the desired duration of sleep is achieved.

There are many forms of relaxation techniques and disciplines of alternative medicine that can be used to promote relaxation, reduce anxiety and help prepare an individual for sleep. These techniques capitalize upon the close harmony between the mind and body which both respond to the environment. Modern research has gone beyond the idea that the mind and body act together as the "mindbody" or "bodymind". It is believed that humankind cannot only train their mind and body to be under a major degree of self-control, but the deepest body processes involving the control of organ functions, e.g. kidney function, gastrointestinal function, etc., can also be subject to self-control. This potential control of the body viscera (body organs) has been called "Visceral Learning" by Gerald Jonas, a staff writer for The New Yorker magazine.

Gerald Jonas has explored techniques, such as yoga, principles of Zen philosophy and transcendental meditation, and their involvement in self-control of body functions. In his book entitled, "Visceral Learning," Gerald Jonas relates the experience of Japanese and American researchers who have studied brain wave patterns in Zen meditators, Indian yogis and healthy volunteers engaged in transcendental meditation. These experiments show the occurrence of special psychological states, where individuals can achieve a status of being both relaxed and awake. In these states, individuals are relatively undisturbed or undistracted by environmental happenings. It seems that meditation can result in a circumstance where an individual can be awake, but where body metabolism and inner body functions are somewhat quiescent.

Altering the Autonomic Nervous System

One important observation is the ability of different forms of meditation to both "relax" the brain and also suppress activity in what is called the "autonomic nervous system." When stimulated, the autonomic nervous connections cause "flight, fright and fight" responses, as though the body is responding to threats or challenging events in the environment. The "flight, fright and fight" syndrome is a fundamental basis of stress and anxiety. It is thought that continuous stimulation of the body in this manner causes many diseases, such as high blood pressure, coronary heart disease and cancer. Meditation can produce a state that is the antithesis (complete opposite) of the body arousal called the "flight, fright and fight" syndrome.

Readers are encouraged to examine alternative medicine strategies for the promotion of relaxation as preparation for good sleep. Other useful alternative medicine approaches to help promote sleep include: posture therapy (Alexander Technique), aromatherapy, biofeedback, Chiropractic techniques, color therapy, hydrotherapy, hypnosis, pattern therapy, reflexology, Shiatsu and sound therapy.

Subjective Insomnia

Recent studies in sleep clinics seem to indicate that many people who claim that they cannot sleep may be engaged in deceptive thinking. These studies show that about one half of all people who complain of insomnia are getting more sleep than they think. This situation is called "subjective insomnia." Such people may believe that it takes them hours to go to sleep, but many are actually falling asleep within matters of minutes. This situation of subjective insomnia is clearly quite common and it reinforces the importance of keeping a sleep journal. Keeping a regular record of sleep patterns and associative events can assist greatly in both the physicians' and patients' understanding of sleep patterns. Such journals should be kept for a couple of weeks or more and information in these records can be expanded by reports from sleeping partners or family members. Just keeping a small writing pad at one's bedside and jotting down events or thoughts can be quite revealing in many ways!

Stressful Life Events

Temporary insomnia is often linked to day-to-day events that can produce stress that is obvious or stress that is unexpected and passes unrecognized. Psychiatrists and behavioral scientists have expanded the original work of the psychiatrist, Dr. T.H. Holmes, who attempted to give a rating of stressful life events. Dr. Holmes described certain events on a scale from most stressful to least stressful. What many individuals do not recognize is that even positive events in life can cause significant degrees of stress. While most people recognize difficulties with the law, divorce and job loss as quite stressful, fewer individuals are likely to acknowledge the stress caused by becoming richer, having a new baby in the family, engaging in great personal achievements or even going on vacation.

It is a sad situation when hardworking people suffer adverse consequences from vacations because they have interrupted their "workaholic patterns." It may be that such people are covering up unresolved conflicts by working hard; and the moment that work stops, the mind starts rehashing unresolved problems. Certain holidays, such as Christmas, are times for both excitement or joy and "fits of the blues." Perhaps it is normal to expect some temporary disruption in sleeping patterns with certain life events or certain times in one's life.

The Natural Way to Healthy Sleep

We live in an age of great belief in medical miracles or "quick-fixes," but getting a good night's sleep should not be tantamount to "popping a drug" to help one sleep. I reiterate that lifestyle and behavioral changes are first-line approaches which can be assisted by the use of natural agents that provide nutritional support to promote healthy sleep. My strong belief is that drugs for sleeping should be used only when other approaches have failed. This opinion is supported by the recorded decline in the use of prescription sleep drugs over the past 30 years. This decline in the use of prescription hypnotic drugs shows that a body of opinion has emerged in medical practice where pharmaceuticals for sleep are perceived as possessing several disadvantages and limitations.

The use of prescription sleep drugs was at its highest in the mid 1970s, when a large number of new drugs to help sleep became available. About 30 years ago there were up to 40 million prescriptions per year written for sleeping pills, whereas today the number is perhaps around 10 million to 15 million prescriptions per year. What has increased is self-medication with drugs for sleep. The market for over-the-counter (OTC) sleeping drugs in the U.S. is huge, where as many as 25 million Americans purchase OTC drugs, usually of the antihistamine type, to help induce sleep.

One could argue strongly that OTC sleeping drug use is a major public health concern given the potential common side effects of these OTC drugs. Unfortunately, the documentation of the side effects of OTC drugs depends largely upon self reporting of adverse effects. Therefore, it is not known how damaging OTC sleeping drugs really are! Clearly, there is a major incentive to seek simpler, gentler and natural alternatives to drugs to promote sleep. These notions are the basis of the "Sleep Naturally Plan."

REFERENCES

Books and Articles

Albert K, *Get a Good Night's Sleep*, Simon and Schuster, NY, 1996

Aspects of Anxiety, J.B. Lippincott Co., Philadelphia, 1965

Barker LR et al, *Principles of Ambulatory Medicine Fourth Edition*, Williams and Wilkins, Baltimore, 1994

Braverman ER, *The Healing Nutrients Within*, Basic Health Publications, Inc., North Bergen, NJ, 2003

British Herbal Pharmacopoeia, British Herbal medicine Association, UK, 1996

Brown DJ, *Herbal Prescriptions for Better Health*, Prima Publishing, California, 1996

Blumenthal M et al, *Herbal Medicine*, Integrative Medicine Communications, 2000

Castleman M, *The Healing Herbs*, Bantam Books, New York, 1995

Crawley J, *The Biorhythm Book*, Virgin Publishing, London, 1996

Fugh-Berman A, *Alternative Medicine: What Works*, Odonian Press, Arizona, 1996

Holt S, *Combat Syndrome X, Y and Z…*, Wellness Publishing, Newark, NJ, 2002

Holt S, *Miracle Herbs*, Carol Publishing, Secaucus, NJ, 1998

Holt S, *Natural Ways to Digestive Health*, M. Evans and Company Inc. New York, 2000

Holt S, *The Antiporosis Plan*, Wellness Publishing, Newark, NJ, 2002

Holt S, *The Natural Way to a Health Heart*, M. Evans and Company, New York, 1999

Holt S, Stewart IC, Dixon JM, Elton RA, Taylor RV, Little K. *Alcohol and the emergency service patient.* British Medical Journal 281:638-40, 1980.

Holt S, Skinner HA, Israel Y. *Identification of alcohol abuse. II.*

Clinical and laboratory indicators. Canadian Medical Association Journal 124(10):1279-94, 1981.

Holt S. *Tackling the alcohol problem: the case for secondary prevention.* Journal of the South Carolina Medical Association 85(12):582-4, 1989.

Holt S. *Identification and intervention for alcohol abuse.* Journal of the South Carolina Medical Association 85(12):554-9, 1989.

Holt S. *Management of gastroesophageal reflux disease - Part I.* Internal Medicine for the Specialist 11, 11:100-106, 1990.

Holt S. *Management of gastroesophageal reflux disease - Part II.* Internal Medicine for the Specialist 11, 12:57-63, 1990.

Holt S, Saleeby G. *Gastric mucosal injury induced by anti-inflammatory drugs* (NSAIDs). Southern Medical Journal 84, 3:355-360, 1991.

Holt S, Powers RE. *Contemporary concerns about acid-suppressing medications.* Current Opinion in Gastroenterology 6:947-951, 1990.

Holt S, *Phytoestrogens for Healthier Menopause.* Journal of alternative and Complementary Therapies. June 1997.

Johns Cupp M and Tracy TS, *Dietary Supplements*, Humana Press, Totowa, NJ, 2003

Jonas G, *Visceral Learning*, Viking Press, New York, 1972

Kales A MD, *Sleep Physiology and Pathology*, A Symposium, J.B. Lippincott Co., Philadelphia, 1969

Kronenberg F and Fugh-Berman A, *Complementary and Alternative Medicine for Menopausal Symptoms: A Review of Randomized, Controlled Trials*, Annals of Internal Medicine, Vol 137 No 10, 2002

Levine SA and Kidd PM, *Antioxidant Adaptation*, Allergy Research Group, California, 1986

Lewis AE and Clouatre D, *Melatonin and the Biological Clock*, Keats Publishing, Connecticut, 1996

Leyden-Rubenstein LA, *The Stress Management Handbook*, Keats Publishing, Connecticut, 1998

Mayell M, *Off-the-Shelf Natural Health*, Bantam, New York, 1995

Murray MT, *The Healing Power of Herbs*, Prima Publishing, California, 1992

Reavley N, *Vitamins etc*, Bookman Press, Melbourne, 1998

Rosenfeld I, *Dr. Rosenfeld's Guide to Alternative Medicine*, Random House, New York, 1996

Schrader C, Beyond 50: *The Road Ahead*, Doubleday, New York, 1999

Schwarzbein D and Deville N, *The Schwarzbein Principle*, Health Communications, Florida, 1999

Skinner HA, Holt S, Allen BA, Haakonson NH. *Correlation between medical and behavioural data in the assessment of alcoholism.* Alcohol Clinical and Experimental Research 4:371-7, 1980.

Skinner HA, Holt S, Israel Y. *Identification of alcohol abuse. I. Critical issues and psychosocial indicators for a composite index.* Canadian Medical Association Journal 124(9):1141-52, 1981.

Skinner HA, Holt S. *Early intervention for alcohol problems.* Journal of the Royal College of General Practitioners 33:787-91, 1983.

Small M, Our Babies, *Ourselves*, Anchor Books, 1998

The Complete Book of Natural and Medicinal Cures, The Editors of Prevention Magazine Health Books, Berkley Books, New York, 1996

The Medicine Show, The Editors of Consumer Reports Books, Consumers Union, NY, 1980

Tyler VE, *Herbs of Choice*, Pharmaceutical Products Press, New York, 1994

Tyler VE. *The Honest Herbal*, Pharmaceutical Products Press, New York, 1993

Ward J, *Dreams and Omens*, Foulsham's "New" Popular Handbook, W. Foulsham and Co. Ltd., London, UK, circa 1950

Whitaker J, *Dr. Whitaker's Guide to Natural Healing*, Prima Publishing, California, 1995

Wiley T.S. and Formby B, *Lights Out*, Simon and Schuster, NY, 2000

Web Sites

www.asda.org
American Sleep Disorders Association

www.nih.gov
National Institutes of Health

www.nsc.org
National Safety Council

www.nhtsa.gov
U.S. National Highway Traffic Safety Administration

www.niaaa.nih.gov
National Institute on Alcohol Abuse and Alcoholism

www.sleepfoundation.org
National Sleep Foundation

www.sleepnet.com
SleepNet

www.stanford.edu
Stanford University Center for Narcolepsy

www.talkaboutsleep.com
Talk About Sleep

www.thinkquest.org
Think Quest

ABOUT THE AUTHOR

Stephen Holt, M.D. is a board-certified internist and gastroenterologist. He is an industry best-selling author from New York. Dr. Holt is a frequent guest lecturer at scientific meetings and a popular media expert on therapeutics.

OTHER BOOKS BY THE AUTHOR:

Skinner HA, Holt S, The Alcohol Clinical Index, Addiction Research Foundation, Toronto, 1993

Holt S, Soya for Health, Mary Ann Liebert Publishers, NY, 1996

Holt S and Comac L, Miracle Herbs, Carol Publishing, NJ, 1997

Holt S and Barilla J, The Power of Cartilage, Kensington Publishers, NY, 1998

Holt S, The Sexual Revolution, ProMotion Publishing, San Diego, California, 1999

Holt S, The Natural Way to a Healthy Heart, M. Evans Inc., 1999 (second printing 2002)

Holt S, The Soy Revolution, Dell Publishing, Random House, NY, NY, 1999 (third printing 2002)

Holt S, Natural Ways to Digestive Health, M. Evans Inc., 2000 (second printing 2002)

Holt S and Bader D, Natures Benefit For Pets, Wellness Publishing, Newark, NJ, 2001

Holt S, Natures Benefit From Coral Calcium: Sorting Science from Speculation, Wellness Publishing, Newark, NJ, 2002, First edition; 2003 Second edition

Holt S, The Antiporosis Plan, Wellness Publishing, Newark, NJ, 2002

Holt S, Combat Syndrome X, Y and Z, Wellness Publishing, Newark, NJ, 2002

Holt S, Digestion, Wellness Publishing, Newark, NJ, 2003

Holt S, Wright J, Syndrome X Nutritional Factors, Wellness Publishing, Newark, NJ, 2003

Holt S, The MenoPlan, Wellness Publishing, Newark, NJ, 2003

Dr. Holt's books are available in major bookstores, fine health food stores and on the Internet at www.wellnesspublishing.com.

Index

Accidents, 13, 17-18, 48, 61, 74, 79, 94
Acid reflux, 38-39
Adaptogenic substances, 8, 111
Advanced sleep phase syndrome, 75
Alcohol, 38, 45, 62, 84, 91, 93, 96, 100, 105, 113, 119-122, 124
Alexander technique, 84, 115
Alternative medicine, 2, 7, 26, 89, 106, 114-115, 119-121
Ambien, 79, 83
Amnesia, 79
Andropause, 83
Antihistamines, 26, 77-78, 93-94
Anxiety, 10, 22, 25, 27, 62, 64-65, 79-81, 83, 88, 92, 95, 99, 102-106, 111, 113-115, 119
Arousal disorders, 66, 73
Ashwagandha, 98, 102-103
Attention Deficit Disorder, ADD, 62

Bacteria, 38, 55-56
Barbiturates, 78-79, 100, 108
Bedroom, 13, 22, 27, 45, 81-82, 93
Beds and mattresses, 84
Bedtime hassles, 64
Behavior modification, 23, 70, 80-81, 84, 111-112
Benzodiazepines, 26, 78-79, 100-101, 107
Biological clock, 22, 40, 52, 120
Biorhythms, 19, 43-44
Body posture, 85-86
Botanicals, 10, 78, 91, 95, 101
Brain, 7, 16, 18-20, 25, 27-29, 32-36, 38, 40, 50-52, 54-57, 59, 61, 63, 65, 67, 74, 89, 99, 101, 107, 109, 114-115

Caffeine, 45, 62, 91-92, 96, 100, 113
Cancer, 42, 57-58, 72, 76, 87, 115
Catnip, 104-105
Central nervous system, 26, 28, 33, 35, 41, 48, 68, 103
Chamomile, 98, 101-102
Chiropractic medicine, 84
Cholesterol, 18, 30, 42, 57, 68, 70, 88, 109
Circadian Oscillator, 48
Circadian Rhythm, 16, 34, 40, 44, 47-48, 53, 74-75, 96
Continuous positive pressure to the airways, CPAP, 68
Cranial Electrical Stimulation, 8, 89

Daylight, 41-42, 107
Deep sleep or REM, 52
Delayed sleep phase syndrome, 75
Delirium, 93
Delta sleep, 19, 49-52
Dementia, 94
Depression, 17, 25, 42, 44, 62, 80, 89, 106
Diabetes mellitus, 17, 72, 76, 109
Dietary supplements, 2, 5, 23, 26, 64, 69-71, 80, 83, 88, 94, 98-99, 120
Diet, 5, 68, 70-72, 91, 109-110, 113
Dreams, 32, 34-37, 53-54, 60,

121
Drowsiness, 16-17, 56, 79, 93, 105
Drug abuse, 16, 79, 89
Drugs, 1-2, 7, 9, 13-14, 18, 22, 26, 29, 38, 46, 52, 62, 64, 68-71, 77-80, 84, 87, 89-91, 93-98, 100-101, 108, 111-113, 116-117, 120

Electroencephalographic, EEG recordings, 19
Emotional cycle, 44
Ephedra (ma huang), 69
Ephedra alternatives, 70
Estrogen, 57-58, 87
Excessive daytime sleepiness, 16, 24, 73, 79
Exercise, 22, 26, 41, 45, 61, 70-71, 80-81, 95, 109-110, 113

First-line options, 9, 23, 31, 111
Flight, fright and fight syndrome, 115
Folic acid, 98, 109-110
Food allergies, food intolerance, 92
Free radicals, 110
Freud S, 35, 44
Fugh-Berman A, 119-120

Gastroesophageal reflux disease, GERD, 38
Glaucoma, 94
Grogginess, 94

Hangover, 15, 25-26, 78-79, 93-94, 100-101, 104, 107
Healthy sleep, 1-2, 9-10, 13-14, 18-19, 22-24, 26, 31, 34, 38, 43, 45-46, 49, 54, 76, 83, 91, 95, 116
Heart disease, 17, 19, 42-43, 57, 76, 109-110, 115
Herbs, 7, 10, 26, 77-78, 83, 91, 95, 100, 103-104, 119-121, 124
High blood cholesterol, 18, 30, 42, 68, 70, 88, 109
High blood pressure, 18, 42, 68, 70, 73, 88, 109, 115
Holt S, 7-8, 18, 38, 43, 55, 57, 70, 72, 88, 119-121, 124
Homeostatic mechanisms, 48
Hops, 98, 105-106
Hormone replacement therapy, HRT, 87
Hormones, 30, 39, 41, 43, 50, 52, 55-59, 75, 87, 95
Hours of sleep, 18, 21, 25, 33, 42-43, 49, 53, 63, 113
Hydroxytryptophan, 8, 98
Hypercholesterolemia, 70
Hypertension, 30, 70-71
Hypnotoxin, 39
Hypocretin, 59
Hypoglycemia, 72

Insomnia, 1, 9, 13-18, 21-27, 47, 61-62, 65, 69, 72, 77, 79-82, 89-92, 95-96, 99, 108, 110-116
Insulin resistance, 18, 42-43, 68, 70, 88
Intellectual cycle, 44
Interleukins, 38, 56
Internet, 23, 25, 53, 124

Jet lag, 75-76, 107-108
Jonas G, 120

Kronenberg F, 120

Learning, 25, 28, 50, 53-54, 63, 89, 114, 120

Leg discomforts, 66
Lemon balm, 98, 104
Lifestyle change, 9, 23, 26, 67, 78, 90, 111-112
Light and dark, 21, 40-41, 49, 107
L-tryptophan, 106
Low Carbohydrate Diet Facilitator, 72

Magnesium, 98, 109
Melatonin, 8, 43, 52, 55-56, 59, 75, 83, 95, 97-98, 106-108, 110, 120
Memory, 17, 21, 25, 36, 53, 63, 67, 75, 79, 82
Menopause, 30, 58, 81, 83, 87-88, 104, 120
MenoPlan, 88, 124
Milk, 26, 45, 61, 92

Napping, 21, 29, 45
Natural remedies, 5, 7
Niacin, 98, 109
Night terrors, 53
Nocturnal food cravings, 72
Nocturnal teenagers, 25

Obesity, 18, 30, 42, 58, 68, 70-71, 73, 88
Oculogram, 19
Osteoporosis, 94, 107, 109-110
Over-the-counter drugs, 7, 52, 77, 93, 111, 117

Parasomnias, 66, 73
Passionflower, 98, 103-104
Penile erections, 39, 49
Physical cycle, 44
Plants, 33-34, 105
Polycystic Ovary Syndrome, PCOS, 72
Poor sleep, 7-8, 13, 17, 22, 25, 30-31, 52, 62, 69, 76, 82, 85, 87, 92, 112
Premenstrual syndrome, PMS, 58, 88
Progesterone, 57-58, 87
Probiotics, 55
Psychiatric disorders, 53, 108

Recovery sleep, 22
Relaxation techniques, 112, 114
Restless leg syndrome, 66, 73, 92, 99

Seasonal Affective Disorder, 44
Self-medication, 26, 99, 117
Simple sugars, 70-72
Skullcap, 98, 103, 105
Sleep aids, 3, 46, 77, 80, 89
Sleep apnea, 9, 15-16, 46, 65, 67-70, 76, 113
Sleep Centers, 9, 13, 60, 63, 83-84, 90
Sleep disorders, 8-9, 15-18, 26, 30-32, 39, 47, 52, 64-66, 70, 72-73, 76, 79-80, 82, 84, 91, 93-96, 112, 122
Sleep deprivation, 7, 16-17, 21-22, 25, 28, 30-31, 33, 38, 40-43, 45, 47, 55, 57-58, 61-62, 73, 81, 88
Sleep history, 14, 84, 96
Sleep in animals, 21
Sleep in elderly, 21, 23, 45, 52, 73, 83
Sleepiness scale, 24
Sleep journal, 45, 115

Sleeplessness, 9, 13, 17, 28-29, 38, 47, 57, 61, 69, 76, 81, 96, 102
Sleep Naturally Plan, 1, 3, 11, 23-24, 80-81, 83, 99, 112, 117
Sleep Number Bed, 85
Sleep research, studies, 34
Sleep-wake cycles, 40
Sleep-talking, 50, 52
Sleepwalking, 19, 39, 46, 51, 54, 66, 73-74, 113
Snoring, 15-16, 45, 52, 67
Stages of sleep, 19, 25, 34, 49-50, 52-53, 56, 63
Stress, 22, 25, 42, 56-58, 61, 64, 75, 78, 92, 94-96, 99-100, 102, 104-105, 107, 109-111, 113, 115-116, 120
Substance abuse, 16-17, 22, 29, 65, 95-96
Sudden Infant Death Syndrome, SIDS, 85
Suprachiasmatic nuclei, 40
Syndrome X, 17-18, 30, 42-43, 57-58, 68, 70-73, 88, 119, 124
Synergy, 7, 97, 108

Time zones, 22, 40, 75
Toxins, 32, 55, 86-87
Triazolam, 79

Valerian, Valerian root, 98-100
Valium, 101
Vitamins, 8, 109-110, 121

Wakefulness, 18, 20-21, 32, 34, 40, 47-48, 50-51, 53, 56, 59, 66, 79, 81-82, 92, 113
Weight control, 30, 41, 57, 67, 69-71, 113

Yoga, 27, 114

Zanasec, 38
Zen, 114
Zolpidem, 79